HIPPOCRATES WEEPS

HIPPOCRATES WEEPS

An Indictment of Changes for the American Health-Care System

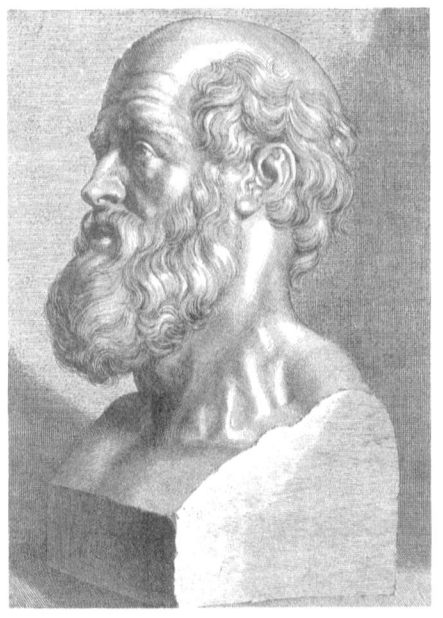

J. WILLIAM EVANS, MD

iUniverse, Inc.
Bloomington

Hippocrates Weeps
An Indictment of Changes for the American Health-Care System

Copyright © 2012 by J. William Evans, MD

All rights reserved. No part of this book may be used or reproduced by any means, graphic, electronic, or mechanical, including photocopying, recording, taping or by any information storage retrieval system without the written permission of the publisher except in the case of brief quotations embodied in critical articles and reviews.

The information, ideas, and suggestions in this book are not intended as a substitute for professional medical advice. Before following any suggestions contained in this book, you should consult your personal physician. Neither the author nor the publisher shall be liable or responsible for any loss or damage allegedly arising as a consequence of your use or application of any information or suggestions in this book.

iUniverse books may be ordered through booksellers or by contacting:

iUniverse
1663 Liberty Drive
Bloomington, IN 47403
www.iuniverse.com
1-800-Authors (1-800-288-4677)

Because of the dynamic nature of the Internet, any web addresses or links contained in this book may have changed since publication and may no longer be valid. The views expressed in this work are solely those of the author and do not necessarily reflect the views of the publisher, and the publisher hereby disclaims any responsibility for them.

Any people depicted in stock imagery provided by Thinkstock are models, and such images are being used for illustrative purposes only.

Certain stock imagery © Thinkstock.

ISBN: 978-1-4697-7700-9 (sc)
ISBN: 978-1-4697-7701-6 (hc)
ISBN: 978-1-4697-7702-3 (e)

Library of Congress Control Number: 2012903075

Printed in the United States of America

iUniverse rev. date: 03/02/2012

Quotes from Hippocrates

The chief virtue that language can have is clearness, and nothing detracts from it so much as the use of unfamiliar words.

Wherever the art of medicine is loved, there is also the love of humanity.

There are in fact two things, science and opinion; the former begets knowledge, the later, ignorance.

Whenever a doctor cannot do good, he must be kept from doing harm.

Cure sometimes, treat often, comfort always.

Everything in excess is opposed to nature.

Make a habit of two things: to help or at least to do no harm.

To my family, who put up with my love affair with medicine, which at times took away from quality activities with them. Also, to my physician colleagues, who for the most part shared a desire to do something for humanity, and for whom I have deep respect and affection. Finally, in memory of my mother, Edna Evans, who shattered my professional basketball ambitions with the statement, "That's nice, Bill, but be sure and do something for humanity."

Contents

Preface xi
My Family's Influences 1
Medical School Training 7
The Medical Oaths 14
The Polluted Oaths: The Profession's Shame 19
My Internship and Residency 23
My Mentors 28
Personalities and Medical Training 35
My Military Service and Early Practice 38
Corporate Medicine 47
Insurance's Invasion into the Practice of Medicine 64
Medicine's Contribution to the Mess 67
Managed Competition 75
My Personal Experiences with HMO Intrusion 85
My Professional Experiences with HMO Intrusion 94
Effects of Changes on Health-Care Professionals 103
Problems in Caring for the Medically Indigent 106
Physician Turned "Enemy of the People" 110
Middlemen: HMOs, IPAs, PPOs, Etc. 113
Personal Practice Changes 118
Brain Drain and Loss of Resources 132
The Solutions 138
Epilogue 143
Endnotes 147
Suggested Reading 151

Preface

Maturation and aging involve learning to live with compromise, dealing with disillusionment when ideals are frequently not obtained, and discovering that others' agendas are usually, consciously or unconsciously, motivated by personal gain. For me, as a physician, this process has taken place as I've watched the most recent attempts at health-care reform unfold, seen self-serving interests take control, and felt the frustration of trying to do my best to serve my patients, often only to have my efforts thwarted by an unsympathetic community—specifically, the insurance-controlled health industry. All of these experiences have driven me to try to put to paper my synopsis of the current crisis in medicine and the perversion of medical ethics.

The idea that one man's experience and chronology of the evolution of his professional career may have meaning to others and may influence the direction of a nation to provide properly for the health care of its citizens may be the height of arrogance, narcissism, stupidity, or some combination of all three. However, my experience can, at least, be an illustration of the current crisis that is closer to the truth than what is currently being presented in the general press. After all, as John Steinbeck wrote, "There are those among us who live in rooms of experience that you and I can never enter."

As a physician with a specialty in general and child psychiatry, I have lived in a room of experience that the average American has never entered; thus, I believe I am in a distinctive position to share much of the frustration that is beginning to pervade the experience of all doctors of medicine. As a teenager, I read Ibsen's *Enemy of the People*,[1] and I recall a statement by the central character, Dr. Stockmann: "Oh, I'm well aware this is small scale compared with a lot of other places." I used to feel that my experience was small-scale compared to the experiences of others, but over time, as I compared my experiences with those of my colleagues, both in my community and around the country, I came to believe that my perceptions of the medical care in this country contained a universal truth and, as such, could be cause for universal alarm.

In regard to this universal truth, Ibsen also wrote, "People want only special revolutions, in externals, in politics, and so on. However, that is just tinkering. What really is called for is a revolution of the human mind." Likewise, the political dancing that is now going on in this country, in regard to health-care reform, is meaningless. We need a revolution in thinking and compassion, one that focuses on the health of our entire nation and does not whittle off some individuals from access to medical care because they are poor, are minorities, have sexual orientations different from those of the majority, are developmentally disabled, have no political clout, or work in small businesses. We need a revolution of enlightenment that results in our focusing on providing universally for the health care of all of our citizens.

I write about my experiences with a great deal of trepidation, and with fear that I will in some way antagonize the powers that be, who can control my life professionally, personally, and socially. I don't see myself as an oppositional personality trying to stir a pot of controversy. All my life, however, I've had an extreme dislike for unfairness and for self-serving people, and when they intrude on my life or on the lives of people I care about, I find it intolerable. Therefore, I am prepared to draw flack for my public reflections and have girded myself accordingly. As Dr. Stockmann says in *Enemy of the People*, "A man should never put on his best trousers when he goes out to battle for freedom and truth."

Because of my experiences, I feel like the character in *Broadcast News*, who shouts out the window, "I'm mad as hell, and I'm not going to take it anymore!" But I want to do more than impotently shout. I want to stimulate critical thinking.

I also want to finish my career as a physician treating people in the manner I was taught, keeping the patient's needs and the well-being of the individual first, and not being subsumed by the group; it would help fulfill a carefully embedded dictate from my mother that, beyond anything else in my professional calling, I need to "do something for humanity."

Today, unfortunately, the fulfillment of that dictate and the maintenance of trust between patient and physician appear to be at an all-time low. When I began practicing, I felt I could treat people to the best of my ability, and, unless I was not meeting the standard set by my peers, would not be condemned for it. Yes, that was a gullible, naïve time in medicine, but it was better than what exists today.

Therefore, this book is about the attempts of society, politics, and the insurance industry to force the deterioration of medical ethics, as well as the invasion of business into the privileged, confidential patient-physician relationship. I express my outrage at the current trends in medicine and the need for a dramatic change in the direction of health-care delivery. Further, I discuss these problems with our medical system against the backdrop of my personal experience, which I believe will help readers understand on a more personal level how far our medical system has fallen from the ideal in recent decades.

The Hippocratic Oath is a noble tradition that embodies the values held universally by all physicians. These values are being eroded, ignored, minimized, and relegated to an obscure place in history. Hippocrates would weep to see the present application of his work. Physicians need to step forward to reaffirm the values of the oath.

My Family's Influences

I needed help with speech as a child, so my parents had me spend time over at Dr. Cheatle's house, a neighbor and family friend. He was a large man, but very kind, and I remember him lying in his bed with a smile on his face, always with a warm, comforting word for me. I never knew why at the time, but later I found out he had been put on bed rest for kidney disease.

"Come on in, Bill," he'd say. "Climb up here, and let's get to work."

A pudgy two-year-old with big, thick glasses, I would climb up on Dr. Cheatle's massive chest and sit perched there, while he carefully and slowly pronounced one word after another and had me repeat them.

"Poe-tae-toe," he would say.

"Potato," I would repeat.

"Toe-mae-toe."

"Tomato."

"Cahl-ih-flow-er."

"Cauliflower."

I don't recall how many weeks or months this went on, but I know this kindly man with the patience of a saint spent every weekday morning with me, for several hours, just repeating words and teaching me to say them correctly.

Dr. Cheatle was in the position to help me learn to speak correctly because he had the time. Ill with kidney disease, he had been told he had little time to live. At that time, sixty-five years ago, his physicians had thought that bed rest was the only treatment likely to help. His prognosis was grim, but the human spirit frequently beats the odds, and, in Doc Cheatle's case, he recovered, returned to his practice, and lived another twenty years.

This was my first introduction to a doctor, a physician, and a healer. The ingredients that made up this man were a sense of power, kindness, caring, patience, and dedication to a task, and that image of him never left me. Those integrated human characteristics stuck in my memory as the very likeness of what a medicine man or woman should be. Would I have learned to talk without his help? Surely. Would I have become a physician without it? Possibly. But would I have the sense of how a physician should be devoted, dedicated, and committed to people? Not likely.

Other Experiences That Shaped My Perception

Probably the earliest and most basic experience unconsciously pushing me toward medicine was my need, as a child, for very thick glasses. My visual problems were unknown at birth, but when I was about two, the diagnosis of astigmatism and hyperopia (farsightedness) were made, and I received my first pair of glasses. They were a godsend to me. My mother told me that once outside the ophthalmologist's office, I got down on my hands and knees to examine the cracks in the sidewalk, and picked up leaves to see them up close. I had not seen the fine images of the world until that time; only gross outlines and fuzzy representations. My glasses thus became important to me. Often, I would sleep with them on my face, refusing to take them off for fear that if

I woke up unexpectedly and needed them, I wouldn't be able to find them.

I believe my unusually thick glass caused some people to assume I must be defective in other ways, for example, intellectually or athletically. In fourth grade, my teacher, Mr. Young, told my mother that, at the beginning of the school year, he had thought I would be "slow" due to my appearance and shy temperament.

"Only after time," he told her, "seeing that every time I asked Bill a question, he'd give me the right answer, did I realize he had a really good mind."

I was also a better-than-average athlete, but it took time for my coaches and classmates to appreciate that. I participated in many sports—baseball and basketball primarily—but often did not have the confidence to try out for a school team and thus to achieve my potential.

Unfortunately for me, my thick glasses internally altered my perception of myself. I thought of myself as ugly and different-looking. I remember, on one occasion, going into a restaurant with my parents, and as we walked by a booth where two elderly women were sitting, I heard one say to the other, "He would be a nice-looking boy if it weren't for those glasses." That and many other similar experiences, minor as they may seem now, insidiously caused me to be self-conscious and lack confidence.

My sophomore year in college, some of that changed when I began wearing contact lenses. My poor vision became less apparent, and others' perceptions of me less skewed. I do recall, with pain, however, an experience during my first few months in college that seemed to be history repeating itself. Colorado College, an excellent small liberal arts institution in Colorado Springs, had a college bowling team. I had become an excellent bowler at my high school in St. Louis, Missouri, the "Bowling Capital of the United States," having spent many hours in practice and winning a number of tournaments. I joined the college team and was immediately recognized as one of the best bowlers in the school.

I took pride in doing well at the sport. On one occasion, I scored exceptionally well, rolling almost a 700 three-game series (900 being the highest possible) and having a high single game of 298 (300 being perfect). At the time, it was the highest game ever bowled in the school's history. I was proud of that, and I do not believe smug. My pride was cut short, however, when a sportswriter for the school paper wrote, "Saucer Eyes Bill Evans rolled a near perfect game at the school bowling alley." Once again, my glasses, and not my accomplishment, had defined me.

Studies have shown that a high number of individuals who enter medicine have been led to do so by heightened anxiety about their health or traumatic medical experiences in childhood. As such, I do not believe that my trips to the ophthalmologist or the procedures done on my eyes or my poor vision in general pushed me toward medicine. Rather, it was my damaged perception of my body's integrity, caused by others' reactions to my glasses.

There were other experiences as well. From age five to age nine, I lived with my family in Germany, where my father, an army officer, was assigned. At age six, not looking where I was going, I ran into the street and was struck by a bicycle. Not realizing the extent of the injury in my left leg, I got to my feet and tried to run, only to have the bone rupture through the skin and crunch into the pavement.

The emergency was extreme, requiring three months of hospitalization, surgeries, meetings with various doctors, and extensive physical therapy and rehabilitation. Again, the process involved contact with many physicians who were kind, caring, committed, dedicated, consistently helpful, and always available when needed.

My perception of what a physician should be was thus forming like an onion, with the core—the initial substance laid down by Dr. Cheatle—being surrounded by layers that followed the same pattern.

Other layers were added over the years: the care given after a broken arm, an accidental overdose of chlorine gas, and after an anaphylactic allergic reaction to penicillin, along with the medical attention given to my brother when he experienced smoke inhalation and almost died. Medical people, in my mind, were helpers. They did not talk about money; they talked about relief of suffering. They made you feel better. Sometimes they did things that had to hurt you up front, but the end result was always a return to health and better functioning. Each step of the way, my perceptions of the honor and purpose within the medical profession was crystallizing.

My Parents' Influence

My father's influence was also extremely significant. As a career army officer, my dad frequently had army physicians under his command. He held them in high regard and always stressed his admiration for their work and dedication. In addition, of all the people I'm aware of on the earth, my father is the most honest and fair man I know.

He'd say, "Bill, I don't care what you've done, but don't ever lie to me. I'll be there for you, for anything, as long as you're truthful with me." His message was very straightforward and clear: always do your best and take care of your responsibilities. His values and the qualities he admired were exceedingly compatible with my ultimate desire to become a physician.

My mother was another large influence, particularly in helping me understand what practicing medicine was really about. She was a very kind and compassionate, extremely intelligent, but unassuming woman, who spent most of her life giving to others, perhaps even in a self-effacing manner. She was trained as a registered nurse and had graduated summa cum laude from Ohio State University.

Occasionally, as a child, I would have discussions with my Mom about what it would be like when I grew up. I recall vividly talking about growing up to be a professional athlete and expressing the fantasies that other children had of power, wealth, or fame. But these fantasies were always colored for me by my mom's relatively constant statement: "It's fine to do anything you want, Son, but be sure you do something for humanity."

Years later, I recognize the impact of that kind of statement. In a diminished way, it certainly narrowed my choices of a career both consciously and unconsciously. After all, what professions are more devoted to helping humanity in a very concrete way than religious vocations or human-service occupations such as those in medicine? Through the normal zigzagging of childhood and adolescent thought, I considered being a minister, a veterinarian, a farmer, a forest ranger, and a number of other occupations, but all were fleeting fantasies.

The people who I felt helped humans the most were physicians. Not so unexpectedly, then, as I found myself trying to decide on a college major, and having an aptitude in science and math, I saw a career in medicine as the most reasonable option, and the one that I would be happy with.

Medical School Training

For my undergraduate degree, I attended Colorado College. I was a good student, a better-than-average athlete, and, eventually, a dormitory counselor. And consistent with the subliminal dictation to "do something for humanity," I was a zoology major with a career headed toward medicine.

For medical school, I attended one of the best in the country—the University of California at San Francisco (UCSF). Medical school was a shock to me. Everyone was smart. Everyone was competitive. Everyone was studious. These students were gifted and talented, but not necessarily kind, helpful, or warm. Further, the acquisition of knowledge was stressed the most, as I was often told, "You'd better learn everything, or you might kill someone."

The First Two Years

Attending a medical school like UCSF clearly could never be categorized as a pleasant experience. During the first two years, there was very little exposure to patient care, but a great deal of exposure to new concepts, extraordinary amounts of memorization, and, frequently, very long hours. It could only be labeled as a baptism of anxiety and intense tribulation.

My fellow classmates and I put in inordinate hours to be sure that we excelled in learning the intricacies of the human body, specifically in anatomy, biochemistry, physiology, microbiology, statistics, pharmacology, and other such classes. After the first few weeks, I had no illusions of excelling or being the first in the class; I just tried to keep up. I had been near the top of my class as an undergraduate, but learned to accept being in the middle of my class in medical school, adhering to the old joke: "What do you call the person who is last in his class in medical school? Doctor."

The mandate was to cure disease; the injunction was to be helpful to patients. Mentors stressed the need for long hours, dedication, thoroughness, and competence. The ethics of medicine were taken for granted, and there was no teaching of fiscal matters. (I would have been floored to hear then how fiscal matters would eventually twist the practice of medicine in this country.) The bottom line: we were all to be healers, academicians, and perhaps researchers, and for this, we would make a decent living.

Competition was fierce. I had come from a small liberal arts school in Colorado and had studied adequately in college but had not had to really put forth the kind of effort that was required of a medical student. At my medical school, there were graduates from Harvard, Stanford, other Ivy League schools, and many from the University of California at Berkeley.

There was a larger percentage of University of California undergraduates in my medical institution since it was a state-supported school, but these students seemed to have needed to fight the hardest and be the most competitive to get into medical school in the first place. In fact, by my assessment, the process of competing to get into medical school had contorted the personalities of this group of first-year medical students from Berkeley. Many of them were extremely obnoxious, if not cutthroat. Some refused to take vacations when the school awarded them to us, preferring to stay at the school and work, hoping to gain an upper hand in the class ranking.

I am a somewhat pragmatic person, probably not as intellectual as some in curiosity, at least from a literary standpoint, and as a result, I am probably not considered by many to be well-rounded. That is, I read, but I do not read constantly. At least, I do not read literature constantly. I read only medicine and psychiatry constantly, and only recently, have begun to read some literature uninvolved with medicine. In medical school, I was confronted by people who were far better readers than I and whose vocabularies were considerably more sophisticated, although some of these individuals may have just used their esoteric vocabularies as a way to impress others.

The first two years were difficult because there was little patient contact. There was a lot to learn, including a completely new language, and the work was hard. There were times I considered dropping out, because I was not certain I wanted to contend with the intensity of the other students. Although I considered myself a relatively competitive person, the egos of these budding physicians, at times, seemed overwhelming. There was definitely a reward for being driven, and as a result, some of my classmates were outright distant, aloof, and unfriendly.

At one point during the first year of medical school, I seriously thought of quitting. Several other students had dropped out, one being my best friend and a fellow who was tremendously engaging and who easily connected with people. In fact, in the first weeks of school, he had been elected our class president. Unfortunately, he did not have the commitment to endless study, and his grades quickly slipped far below those of the bulk of the class. With each individual who left, I further questioned my ability to sacrifice in the way that I was beginning to learn that a physician needed to subjugate other needs to the service of becoming a good physician. When I went to my advisor to discuss dropping out, she had the good sense to talk to me as a caring human being, telling me it would get better and to get my butt back to the books and keep at it.

Gradually, I found my niche. I found others who shared my concern for the lack of exposure to humans, particularly during the first year of medical school. And it was only with the introduction of the patient experience that I started to feel that I had made the right choice.

The Final Two Years

The core experience of my final two years of med school was the exposure to patients, wherein the magnitude of the responsibility of caring for humans became clear. Puzzling illnesses would require me to spend many hours, nights, and bedside time trying to find what was wrong, and trying to help. Still, assisting patients was extremely rewarding. It was challenging and exciting. There was a thrill in actually having diagnosed and helped someone; there was patient gratitude; there was respect from other individuals. And, most of all, there was a sense that I was "doing something for humanity." When dealing with patients and making rounds, I felt exhilarated. I felt compassion. I was thrilled with the prospect of understanding the human being and being able to help with his or her medical problem.

As with most budding infatuations that turn to true commitment and dedication, the early enthusiasm becomes more integrated, balanced by the discovery of less-desirable aspects of the profession. Doctors, like all populations of human beings, are filled with their share of strange personalities; namely, individuals who behave selfishly, over-aggressively, and, at times, insensitively to the people they care for. I remember being appalled at hearing stories by obstetrical residents who held contests to see who could have the most babies named after them. Frequently, they would pick on single, uneducated women, often black, who were naïve to their intentions. They would influence them to either name their babies after them or to give the babies ridiculous names, which they also claimed credit for.

I experienced high anxiety whenever I had to go on rounds with one particular sadistic attending physician, who seemed to delight in ridiculing me in front of my peers, insensitively pointing out how little I really knew. I didn't take it personally, however. There were a few classmates who seemed to pick up one of the nuances of an illness or figure out the more esoteric diseases before the majority of us did, but I recognized that it was tough for all of us and that I wasn't being picked on or singled out. We were all in this together.

There were also moments of humiliation set up by house staff, interns, or residents to make me look like a fool and then get a good laugh at my expense. One such instance, which I remember most vividly, was the time a resident had me prepare a patient awaiting orthopedic surgery. The patient, a male, had already been sedated and needed to be catheterized; that is, I had to place a tube in his penis to drain off urine as it accumulated during the procedure. First, however, the penis needed to be cleansed with soap and water. This washing was done primarily with a swab. Even though the patient is asleep, the cleansing is apparently sexually stimulating and frequently results in the patient obtaining an erection. At the time, however, I was not aware of that fact. And, of course, as luck would have it, the patient did get an erection, at which point, among the entourage of interns, other medical students, nurses, residents, and attending staff standing around, the senior resident looked over at me and said, "Evans, I told you to clean him off, not jack him off." Turning bright red, I finished my preparation while everyone around me got a derisive laugh.

One of my outlets for built-up frustration was the Student Union basketball program. Each medical class year had a team, as did the pharmacy and dental school classes, and different departments in the hospital, (e.g., Internal Medicine, Orthopedics.) I was a better-than-average player, but more important, I was able to channel my life frustrations into aggressive play.

My third and fourth years were all clinical work, all oriented to patients. There was constant supervision by senior and junior staff members, residents, interns, each one looking over my shoulder, judging me, helping me form an appreciation for the magnitude of the task that was patient care. It was also during this time that a hierarchy of suffering in the service of patients seemed to arise: Who could stay up the longest? Who could see the most patients? And, for me, given my personal mandate, who could contribute the most to humanity?

Further Reflections

It has been interesting, over the course of my professional life, to have met and become good friends with many physicians who have reaffirmed how universally difficult medical school was for most of us. In fact, I now believe that many physicians have marginal symptoms of post-traumatic stress disorder related to their training experiences.

Post-traumatic stress disorder has to have certain criteria attached to it for the diagnosis to be considered. First, a person must have experienced an event outside the normal human experience, an event that almost anyone else would find distressing. Second, this event must be persistently re-experienced through distressing recollections, dreams, reminders, or sudden feelings that the event is recurring. There also may be efforts by the sufferer to avoid thoughts or feelings associated with the trauma, an inability to recall an important aspect of the trauma, a highly diminished interest in significant activities in the present, feelings of detachment from others, and the sense of a shortened future. Other symptoms include difficulty sleeping, irritability, problems concentrating, hyperactive vigilance, and an exaggerated startle response.

Through the years, I have treated physician patients or just talked with physician friends, and it is surprising how many of them have enough of these symptoms to meet the criteria for post-traumatic stress disorder. Further, for most, it seemed to be the faculty's lack of caring for their distress during medical school that led to the disorder.

"If you can't cope with the pressure, get out of the profession," seemed to be the standard sentiment of these faculty members. The expected response, if students brought up sleep problems, excessive worry, or recurrent distressing dreams, was that one would be exposed as weak, inadequate, or just not tough enough to be a physician. Because of such insensitivity, no prudent individual would seek help with their symptoms. Instead, he or she would suffer and keep going.

The Medical Oaths

Hippocrates, "the father of western medicine," lived from 460 BC until 370 BC. History portrays him as the paradigm of the ancient physician. He is credited with advancing the systematic study of clinical medicine, integrating the teachings of previous medical schools, and developing prescription practices for physicians by authoring the Hippocratic Oath.[2]

Not all medical schools use the Hippocratic Oath as the standard for ethical direction, but, overall, the oath has been an indispensable fundamental basis for medical ethics and one of oldest sets of ethical guidelines of any profession. Here is the oath, which Hippocrates exacted from students of medicine in his day:

The Hippocratic Oath
I swear by Apollo the Physician and Aesculapius, and Hygiene and Panacea, and all of the gods and goddesses, that according to my ability and judgment, I will keep this Oath and its stipulation—to reckon him who taught me this art equally dear to me as my parents, to share my substance with him, and to relieve his necessities if required; to look upon his offspring in the same pudding as my own brothers,

and to teach them this art if they shall wish to learn it, without fee or stipulation, and that by precept, lecture, and every other mode of instruction, I will impart a knowledge of the art to my own sons and those of my teachers and to disciplines bound by a stipulation and Oath according to the law of medicine, but to none other.

I will follow that system of regimen which according to my ability and judgment, I consider for the benefit of my patients, and abstain from whatever is deleterious and mischievous. I will give no deadly medicine to anyone if asked, or suggest any such counsel; and in like manner, I will not give to a woman a peccary to produce abortion. With purity and with holiness I will pass my life and practice by art. I will not cut a person laboring on the stone, but will leave this to be done by men who are practitioners of this work. Into whatever houses I enter, I will go into them for the benefit of the sick, and I will abstain from voluntary acts of mischief and corruption and, further, from the seduction of females or males, of free men and slaves. Whatever, in connection with my professional practice or not, in connection with it. I see or hear, in the life of men, which are not to be spoken of abroad, I will not divulge, as reckoning, that all such should be kept secret.

While I continue to keep this Oath un-violated, may it be granted to me to enjoy life and the practice of this art, respected by all men, in all times. But should I trespass and violate this Oath, may the reverse be my lot.

Elaborating on Hippocrates, Rabbi Moses ben Maimon, a Jewish philosopher and physician in Egypt who lived from 1135 to 1204, composed a prayer used in graduation ceremonies at many medical schools. The Prayer of Maimonides is as follows:

The Prayer of Maimonides

Thy eternal providence has appointed me to watch over the life and health of Thy creatures. May the love for my art actuate me at all times; may neither avarice nor miserliness, nor thirst for glory, or for great reputation, engage my mind; for the enemies of truth and philanthropy could easily deceive me and make me forgetful of my lofty aim of doing good to Thy children.

May I never see in the patient anything but a fellow creature in pain.

Grant me strength, time, opportunity always to correct what I have acquired, always to extend its domain; for knowledge is immense and the spirit of man may extend indefinitely to enrich itself daily with new requirements.

Today he can discover his errors of yesterday and tomorrow he can obtain a new light on what he thinks himself sure of today. O God, Thou hast appointed me to watch over the life and death of Thy creatures; here am I ready for my vocation and now I turn to my calling.[3]

Further, in 1948, the Second General Assembly of the World Medical Association adopted the Declaration of Geneva. In a number of medical schools today, because of the out-datedness of some aspects of the Hippocratic Oath, the Declaration of Geneva is used in its place. For example, the aspect of Hippocrates's oath that relates to abortion presents a very interesting ethical and philosophical dilemma in present society. Also the narrowness of some aspects of Hippocrates's vows are felt by many to make the Declaration of Geneva a more appropriate ethical affirmation.

Declaration of Geneva

> At the time of being admitted as Member of the Medical Profession, I solemnly pledge myself to consecrate my life to the service of humanity. I will give to my teachers the respect and attitude which is their dues; I will practice my profession with conscience and dignity; the health of my patients will be my first consideration; I will respect the secrets which are confided in me; I will maintain, by all means in my power, the honor and the noble traditions of the medical profession; my colleagues will be my brothers; I will not permit considerations of religion, nationality, race, party, politics or social standing to intervene between my duty and my patients; I will maintain the utmost respect for human life, from the time of conception; even under threat, I will not use my medical knowledge contrary to the laws of humanity. I make these promises solemnly, freely, and upon my honor.[4]

If you canvas most physicians, the understanding of the common bonds between the above oaths would be:

- To treat the patient to the best of one's ability.
- To not allow anything other than what is best for the patient's medical condition to govern the treatment.
- To follow the dictum laid down by Hippocrates, *"Primum non nocere,"* which means, "First, do no harm."

Nurses, our siblings in health care, also depend upon ethical guidance. Nursing has adopted an oath used universally upon capping or graduation as a pledge of the ethical standards of their profession. A committee from the Farrand School of Nursing at Harper Hospital in Detroit, Michigan, formulated the Nightingale Pledge, which reads as follows:

The Nightingale Pledge

I solemnly pledge myself before God and in the presence of this assembly to pass my life in purity and practice my profession faithfully. I will abstain from whatever is deleterious and mischievous. I will not take or knowingly administer any harmful drug. I will do all in my power to maintain and elevate the standards of my profession, and will hold in confidence all personal matters committed to my keeping, and all family affairs coming to my knowledge in the practice of my calling. With loyalty will I endeavor to aid the physician in his work and devote myself to the welfare of those committed to my care.[5]

Physicians and nurses take their respective oaths at the completion of their degree training. It is usually done in a group ceremony during the awarding of the degree.

Regardless of the oath chosen, these oaths are to be taken seriously. I remember being very aware of our recitation of the Hippocratic Oath and its importance to me from a personal ethical perspective, and I believe my fellow students shared my feelings. For me, the basic tenet was to "do no harm." My teachers had always instructed us that fiscal and financial considerations should never come before the proper care of patients. In addition, my medical school training never included discussions about the costs of procedures or care, so, by default, I felt economics to be inconsequential when compared to optimally treating the patient.

My early years of practice were quite consistent with these teachings. I am appalled, however, at how things have changed since.

The Polluted Oaths: The Profession's Shame

In reaction to what is taking place in the practice of medicine today, I have written the following amended "oaths," which I feel more accurately reflect the current realities of the industry. As you read them, you can get a sense of how far the profession has fallen from the ideals expressed in the original oaths. In future chapters, I will go into much more detail about how these polluted oaths come into play.

The Desecrated Hippocratic Oath

I swear by Apollo the Physician and Aesculapius, and Hygiene and Panacea, and all of the gods and goddesses **including insurance companies, health maintenance organizations, preferred provider organizations, and managed care companies,** that according to my ability and judgment, I will keep this Oath and its stipulation—to reckon him who taught me this art equally dear to me as my parents, to share my substance with him, **if he is a part of my provider group,** and to relieve his necessities if required **and if it is economically prudent and meets the requirement of medical necessity**; to look upon his offspring in the same pudding as my own brothers, and to teach them this art if they shall wish to learn it, without fee or stipulation, and that by precept, lecture, and every other mode of instruction, I will impart a knowledge of the art to my own sons and those of my teachers and to disciplines bound by a stipulation and Oath according to the law of medicine **and the insurance industry**, but to none other.

I will follow that system of regimen which according to my ability and judgment, I consider for the benefit of my patients, and abstain from whatever is deleterious and mischievous **unless it is in the best interest of my insurance provider group to do so**. I will give no deadly medicine to anyone if asked, or suggest any such counsel, **and I will give no medicine that is too costly even if it is the best choice for my patient, especially if it has not been made a part of the insurance company's limited pharmaceutical formulary;** and in like manner I will not give to a woman a peccary to produce abortion. With purity and with holiness **and with economic caution** I will pass my life and practice by art. I will not cut a person laboring on the stone, but will leave this to be done by men who are practitioners of this work, **especially if they are approved members of my provider panel and have received proper authorization.** Into whatever houses I enter, I will go into them for the benefit of the sick, **provided they have the appropriate referral form and the insurance-approved primary care physician's sanction,** and I will abstain from voluntary acts of mischief and corruption **unless they economically benefit the insurance industry** and, further, from the seduction of females or males, of free men and slaves **especially the later who surely would not be**

approved for medical care. Whatever, in connection with my professional practice or not in connection with it, I see or hear, in the life of men, which are not to be spoken of a god, I will not divulge as reckoning that all such should be kept secret **except to the insurance industry and its national network of computer data.**

While I continue to keep this Oath un-violated, **although the quality of my care will rarely be recognized,** may it be granted to me to enjoy life and the practice of this art, respected by all men **but especially by the insurance industry, given my economic profile provides cost savings at all times.** But should I trespass and violate this Oath, may the reverse be my lot.

The HMO-Corrupted Prayer of Maimonides

Thy eternal providence has appointed me to watch over the life and **some aspects of the health of a select segment** of Thy creatures. **Although weighing the economic needs of insured patients will likely allow me to deviate from these principles,** may the love of my art **perhaps** actuate me at **some** times; may neither avarice or miserliness, nor thirst for glory or great reputation engage my mind **unless these qualities happen to serve the best interest of the HMOs and insurance companies with whom I contract,** for the enemies of truth and philanthropy could easily deceive me and make me forgetful of my lofty aim of doing good for Thy children.

May I never see in the patient anything but a fellow creature in pain, **unless that affects what is best for the HMO and is judged too costly for its good.**

Grant me strength, time, opportunity always to correct what I have acquired **to the point that economic constraints are observed, always to extend its domain, with an eye toward the economic needs of the group;** for knowledge is immense and the spirit of man extends indefinitely to enrich itself daily with new requirements, **but only if extreme caution is paid to economic viability.**

Today he can discover his errors of yesterday, and tomorrow he can obtain a new light on what he think himself sure of today, **but caution as to economics and resource utilization of the group needs always to be observed.** O God, Thou hast appointed me to watch over the life and death of **some** of Thy creatures; here am I ready for my vocation and now, **if economically credentialed and selected by enough HMOs, regardless of my ability,** I turn to my calling.

My Internship and Residency

My first year as a "real" doctor, or at least as a graduate of medical school, was done at the Good Samaritan Hospital, a private teaching hospital in Phoenix, Arizona. Frequently during my internship, I was given, for the first time, under supervision, total responsibility for the care of patients.

The physicians in practice were my teachers, and many of them taught me well—I will always feel grateful to them. Conversely, a few times, I was also exposed to doctors whose egos and sense of self-aggrandizement or entitlement were so great that I found them almost intolerable to be around. I remember two neurologists, partners, who delighted in having me make rounds with them, just so that I could carry their little black bag. These doctors also put me through a kind of fraternity hazing, in which they constantly reminded me about how little I knew and how important the practicing physician was.

I also remember an OB/GYN who was so idiosyncratic in his practice that, whenever he delivered a baby, he'd have to have a size 7-1/4 glove for one hand and a size 7-1/2 for the other. These were stretchy rubber gloves, and he was delivering newborns, not doing microscopic brain surgery. What was the big deal? In addition, this specialist insisted on using a gold-handled needle when he sutured patients. His technique was exquisite, his patient care was impeccable, but he was exceedingly filled with his own self-importance and not the kind of person one would necessarily pick to be a friend or even to spend time with.

My internship was an extraordinarily demanding year out of my medical training. I was not paid much, and by that time, I had a wife and two children. Halfway through each month, I would volunteer to go on-call because I did not have enough money to buy food and take care of my family. When I was on-call, my family could eat for free at the hospital. Taking call meant long hours and hard work, but it was a way to make ends meet.

I was one of the more sedate members a group of new physicians-in-training who all seemed to have a greater enjoyment for life than those I had encountered at the university. As a group, they were far less serious than the medical students I had studied with before. Because I was one of the few married interns, I did not participate in as many parties as the other interns did. In particular, many of them seemed to engage in a great deal of sexual activity, mostly the single ones, but even some of the married ones. There was also a lot of fraternization between these doctors-in-training and the nurses at the hospital where I interned. In fact, I recall one emergency room nurse who seemed to pride herself on the number of interns she went to bed with each year.

Disillusionment

One of the more disillusioning parts of my internship was the exposure I had to the prejudice and insensitivity held by some medical professionals toward Native Americans, a group of people they considered inferior. I interned in Arizona, and Arizona has a large Native American population. These people are a highly disadvantaged group, often quite poor, and too frequently relegated to the ghettos or reservations where very poor opportunity and human advantage exist. The medical care given to these individuals was, at the time of my internship, segregated. That is to say, there was a hospital specifically for Native Americans, although it was not a mandate that every patient of American Indian heritage go there; in fact, Native Americans were often treated in the general hospital where I interned.

One night after I'd taken care of a number of patients and was very tired, I went to the room where the interns slept in the wee hours of the morning. I fell asleep only to be awakened a little while later by a phone call from the emergency room nurse. She said an ambulance was bringing in a man who'd been in an accident. The extent of his injuries was unknown. The call filled me with trepidation. Whenever a call like this came in, my heart would race, my anxiety level would rise, and I would wait for the worst possible case to be brought through the door. I was still insecure enough in my capabilities that I was sure there would come a day when someone would come in and I wouldn't know what to do. I feared I might not provide the proper medical care and that, if I were the only doctor available, perhaps some individual would die as a result. But in this particular instance, the nurse ended the call with, "Don't hurry; there won't be a problem. It's only an Indian."

I was appalled. I had not encountered that kind of response from a medical person before. It should not have surprised me, though. After all, doctors and nurses are no different than any other group of people. They, like many others, often have prejudices, biases, and an inability to be compassionate to those different from themselves.

It did open my eyes, however unfortunately, to the fact that medical care was selective in how it dealt with different individuals. I became aware that medically indigent patients might receive a different form of attention than those who pay for their care. That racial minorities might receive different care than those who are not racial minorities. That people with different-than-normal sexual orientations might receive inferior care from prejudiced or bigoted medical staff. I have lived in the San Francisco area where there is a large gay population, and I do not believe there is a great deal of discrimination against gay individuals there; however, even among a fairly enlightened medical population, I have known doctors who have refused to care for patients with AIDS, taking the attitude that the disease was somehow deserved by its victims because of their sexual orientations.

Everyone Deserves the Best Medical Care

My experience as an intern taught me that I needed to examine my own prejudices and to be certain that, whenever I encountered someone whose life experience was different from my own, I gave his or her care my best effort. I have remained dedicated to that goal and continue to give the best medical and psychiatric care I can provide to every patient.

The fact is, many individuals in this country do not have health care available to them, and a large portion of those individuals are people who fall into the category of being a minority or just somehow outside the norm of society. These individuals, however, have the same medical rights as any other segment of society. All patients, regardless of their background, sexual orientation, race, or religion, deserve their physician's best efforts, including their greatest expertise and their complete dedication.

It's been enlightening to me to have known colleagues who have worked in prison with murderers, rapists, terrorists, and others who have committed the most heinous of crimes—even people on death row, and those who have tortured and sexually abused children. Many of these doctors and nurses were able to suspend their value judgments and any personal feelings they had toward patients with such backgrounds, and give them extremely competent medical care.

There were exceptions, however. Some physicians would even ridicule their inmate-patients who had psychiatric illnesses or in some other way triggered in the physician a sense of contempt. Such behavior is indefensible. If one is going to work in a situation like a prison, one has to suspend his or her personal feelings and operate only as a physician, dedicated to providing the most competent care possible.

Those physicians who refuse to treat any group of patients with the best possible care should reread the oath they took upon graduating. They swore to help all other human beings—not specific groups of them.

My Residency—Becoming a Good Doctor

As a resident of psychiatry, I learned about mental illness. I learned about the interactions of stress, organic predisposition, and a multitude of other factors, and how those interactions can cause the mind not to work well, incapacitating the individual in a variety of ways.

I also learned that I was good at what I did. I could understand patients, and they understood me. I learned about the relevant medications and used them well. And I was recognized by my fellow residents for my skill. I was becoming a good doctor *and* I was doing something for humanity. *Maybe I could be like Doc Cheatle*, I thought, *and help little kids*. Child psychiatry—that was it. I would be a child psychiatrist.

Most child psychiatrists see some adults, some adolescents, and some children, so you need to be trained first in adult psychiatry and then do a fellowship in child and adolescent psychiatry. And that is exactly what I did.

When I was finished, I thought about Doc Cheatle. He would be proud. My mother and father would be proud too. I was now a physician.

My Mentors

———•◆•———

As a balance to some of the physicians I described earlier, a number of mentors, who I consider myself fortunate to have worked with, have continually renewed my affection for medicine. Several physicians come to mind as individuals who epitomized the values and ideals of medical practice and patient care.

Who is a doctor, a physician, a healer? Is a doctor a wealthy businessman, a humanitarian, or a greedy entrepreneur? The contrasting images are endless, and I think the public as a whole holds a very ambivalent perception of them. Usually people have their own doctors in mind, whom they like, trust, and see as dedicated and compassionate, maybe even seeing them as throwbacks to television doctors, for example, Ben Casey, Dr. Kildare, Marcus Welby, or the myriad of doctors portrayed on *ER* or *Private Practice*. But then there are those *other* doctors we think of— the ones who have money, live in big, nice houses, belong to country clubs, play golf, and drive Porsches, Mercedes, and BMWs; those who have God-complexes, feel they are above people, act condescendingly, and are only interested in maintaining their very well-garnished livings. In real life, I certainly have met the epitome of all of these physician portraits.

After forty years of exposure to medical students, physicians, nurses, and other industry professionals, I can say that I usually feel a kinship and professional liking for them and that I generally respect their work and capabilities. But for now, I want to focus on one man who, for me, has become the ideal of what a successful physician should be.

Dr. Howard Siedler

Several years ago, Dr. Howard Siedler, a friend of mine and a neurologist, became ill while on vacation. He had a seizure and possibly a stroke, and was soon after diagnosed with a brain tumor containing a preponderance of fast-growing cells. He was given a six-months-or-less prognosis. Howard, or Sy, as we called him, had surgery, chemotherapy, and, like any deserving patient, received the best care available at the time. He survived several months beyond his prognosis, but, even with the best medicine available, still died. He died as he had lived, however, with a sense of humor and with dignity.

For me, Howard epitomized a lot of the finer qualities of people in medicine. He was a very quiet man, who, once you got to know him, had tremendous wit and character, and a total lack of arrogance. He was dedicated as well; I remember spending many evening hours seeing patients at the hospital, and frequently Howard would wander in to finish up his day's work. We certainly had camaraderie, and I respected him greatly.

Howard and I would occasionally have lunch together, or sit down during a spare moment for a cup of coffee. Outside of medicine, I did not spend much time with Sy, but I knew he liked nature and had a particular fondness for hiking and gardening. I also knew his daughter, who, at one time, was working toward becoming a mental health clinician and was one of the more excellent staff members that I'd had the pleasure of working with.

Howard had a dry sense of humor and remained unflustered even when things went wrong or when the demands on him had to seem overwhelming. He never lost his cool; he was always professional, always kind, and always a gentleman.

Howard epitomized putting the patient's interest before all else and leaving the business aspect of medicine in a non-priority position, out of the way of the primary doctor-patient relationship. Howard would never refuse to see a patient. He never cared if the patient had money, was medically indigent, or had the right insurance. His priority was to see the person, do the evaluation, and provide the consultation first, and only after that, to collect—or frequently, never collect—whatever fee was available to him.

I admired his dedication. I always knew I could count on him, and I knew that if I needed a neurological consult, he would be there—even for myself. When I injured my neck, he was one of the first doctors I consulted. He also consulted on my eldest son, who is mentally retarded and has a seizure disorder. This, I believe, was one of the keys to Howard's success with patients and colleagues alike. In each relationship he established, Howard also established trust. The other person could always trust that Howard would do his best, uphold his Hippocratic Oath, and know that nothing else mattered.

Of all the good physicians I have known, Howard was not the exception, but, for the most part, the rule. However, he certainly was the finest part of that rule.

I hope that, ultimately, we can return to being a society that allows doctors and patients to have such a sovereign relationship—a relationship in which the business aspect becomes secondary. Although I know many other doctors whose dedication to their clients matches Howard's, I am afraid that, currently, such doctor-client relationships are not the norm. The insurance industry exerts such a pressure on this relationship that the doctor cannot help but to become more concerned about satisfying insurance requirements than about meeting the patient's needs—and the patient gets lost in the process.

Dr. Barry Blackwell

One of my first supervisors was Dr. Barry Blackwell, a British man with a superb sense of humor and training experience very different from my own or any of the other faculty members at the University of Cincinnati, where I completed my psychiatric residency. Dr. Blackwell was a bit of a renegade within the Department of Psychiatry. He was not a psychoanalyst, and certainly not Freudian. He taught me about medications and their usefulness in altering desperate suffering and anguish, or tortured thinking. Of all the things he taught me, however, what I remember most were his admonitions to question the *status quo*, to utilize the scientific method in understanding human beings, and to try to sort out all of the variables that influenced why people behaved the way they did. He did not embrace one approach with religious zeal; rather, he was a scientist. But as a scientist, he helped me understand that a physician needs to be a humanitarian as well as a scientist.

One of the most interesting things I remember during my residency was the fact that I could present one particular case to several different supervisors and get various unique, though perhaps equally valid, perspectives from each of them. All were respected clinicians, but all had different slants on why the patient was behaving as he or she did. Ultimately, I found I would have to rely on building my own clinical experience and convictions. After all, no two humans behaved the same, and no two physicians looking at a human would come to precisely the same conclusion.

It's interesting to note that, in psychotherapy, one of the biggest curative factors, apart from any medications prescribed, is a clinician with warmth, empathy, and the ability to form an alliance with the patient. Over the years, I've found that the intellect of the clinician is also important: the brighter the doctor is, the faster the patient responds and the more benefit he or she achieves from therapy.

Dr. Blackwell's and My Research

In my psychiatric residency at the University of Cincinnati, Dr. Blackwell and I, as well as another resident, carried out what I have always felt to be a very interesting and important research study. It was especially important for my own edification. We were testing the effects of antidepressant medication on analgesic use in a population of patients in a chronic-disease hospital. These patients were housed for literally years in very isolated, desolate units, and needed pain medicine to help with their suffering. They were not psychiatric patients per se, but simply patients with chronic diseases that gave them considerable pain.

In our study, we had two groups of patients—one would receive antidepressant medication, and the other would receive a placebo. Each group would be interviewed weekly by one of the three of us. The weekly interviews were not long—a few minutes to, at most, a half an hour. Our research questions were designed to determine whether the antidepressant would benefit the patients by reducing their voluntary analgesic use.

It was a relatively time-consuming project, but we speculated that many of the chronic-disease patients were also depressed, and that the patients receiving antidepressants would reduce their voluntary analgesic use by reducing their depression. Conversely, we expected that those receiving placebos would continue to require the same amount of analgesic. Since the pain medicines these patients were taking were administered on an as-needed basis, if we were right, then those taking the antidepressants would request their medication less often. Patients were given no indication that their pain medications would have to be reduced in any way; they were told to continue to ask for medicine as they needed it.

Our Findings

The results were surprising: there was a 90 percent reduction in analgesic use by both groups. We had failed to design the research properly by introducing a variable that we had not anticipated. That variable was human contact. Because these patients were living in relative isolation, except for their contact with nursing staff and an occasional visit by the hospital doctor, our entrance into their lives—although seemingly minor to us—proved to be extraordinarily important.

We concluded that, before our project began, the patients may have used their pain, perhaps unconsciously, to establish contact with other human beings. By asking a nurse for medicine, they were able to receive not only contact, but also concern, care, and attention, even if only for a brief moment. During our project, however, these patients had regular interviews with a doctor, and those interviews suddenly became more than sessions for gathering information.

Although disappointed that the results did not confirm our hypothesis, it was very instructive to me to learn that these individuals, who had spent months and sometimes years in a situation that made them feel like outcasts from the world, were so influenced by our weekly interviews that their analgesic use dropped dramatically. It taught me that human beings needed to be dealt with, with compassion. That if the elements of empathy and compassion were introduced into the lives of isolated, despairing people, those elements could far overshadow the use of medication in improving their conditions.[6]

Dr. Blackwell taught me to maintain perspective and a healthy skepticism about what helped patients' conditions improve. He also taught me to look at all the factors involved in a situation instead of jumping to a premature conclusion.

Other Mentors

When I think of all those who have mentored me, reminding me what medicine should be about, many other doctors come to mind. I recall Dr. Charles Carmen from medical school, a superb diagnostician who constantly stressed the need for compassion and for understanding the total patient, rather than seeing each one only as a disease entity. Dr. John Carbone also demonstrated that the total patient was important, emphasizing that the disease was only one facet of what was happening to a person and pointing out that we, as physicians, had to try to comprehend all we could about patients in order to be helpful to them.

In medical school, my first psychiatric mentor was Dr. H. Spencer Bloch, a man who agreed to be my preceptor during an elective time in psychiatry. I had had no experience with psychiatric patients before that; I'd only heard horrendously boring lectures at the Department of Psychiatry at the University of California. Dr. Bloch spent hours helping me understand a few of the intricacies of the human mind, and it was under his tutelage that I decided I wanted to learn more about how the mind worked and what influences molded human behavior. It was after my one-month preceptorship with him that I decided to go into the field of psychiatry.

Finally, my residency program exposed me to many psychiatrists at the University of Cincinnati who each had a great understanding of patients, a great capability to teach, and a great influence on my desire to hone my skills and understanding of what motivated human conduct.

Personalities and Medical Training

Medical training skews a person's personality. In some respects, I think it has changed mine for the worse, and only recently have I tried to recapture some of the characteristics that I liked in myself when I was younger.

This alteration in personality begins with the competition to get into the best medical school, or any medical school for that matter, and it continues, beginning with the very first days of medical training. I recall attending a reception, approximately one week after medical school began. Its purpose was to allow new students to meet with the faculty, deans, assistant deans, department heads, and so on, all of whom formed a receiving line.

When I met the dean, he asked me, "How's it going?"

I responded that I was feeling a little overwhelmed.

"That's good," he said. "We don't want you to feel comfortable. You'll get used to it; it's part of being a physician."

I recall being shocked at the reply, since I had expected more empathy, or at least sympathy—some type of comforting comment. In retrospect, I see his comment as a foreshadowing of the personal sacrifice that would be required of me to become a physician.

Medical training promotes the idea that the more hours you put in, the better doctor you are. On the surface, the idea seems admirable, but, under closer scrutiny, it does not hold water. If I were a patient going into surgery, I would certainly want my surgeon to be well-rested, not someone who had been without sleep for forty-eight hours straight, trying to prove that he or she was the world's greatest doctor. Doctors are rewarded, however, for putting in long hours, seeing countless patients, and neglecting outside interests, which, in many cases, means even their families.

I think a common phenomenon for many physicians is a disillusionment that occurs in midlife, as they realize that the rewards promised from this kind of dedication do not always occur. Yes, there are financial rewards, but there is a great price to pay if they have dedicated themselves so much to work that they find, suddenly, they have grown children about whom they know very little. A number of physicians also have failed marriages—me included—and part of that phenomenon may be due to our marriage to medicine, as opposed to what might be more rewarding commitments to spouses, children, friends, and a well-rounded life.

I believe my first wife had a great deal of trouble with my long hours and the demands of my practice, including a pager that seemed endlessly to interrupt our time together. And as the tension between us increased, I began dedicating more of my time at home to my children. I feel I did a good job of being a father, but, in retrospect, I did a poor job of being a husband. I found it easier to get my reward as a dedicated parent and physician, than as a dedicated husband. I served as president of the PTA, helped lead school task forces, found time to coach my children in sports, and was involved in a lot of their academic work. In addition, two of my three biological children have special needs. My oldest son is mentally retarded, with a seizure disorder. As an adult, he is able to live in a sheltered, semi-supervised setting, but as a child, he required much attention. My youngest son is diabetic, requiring insulin injections and blood-glucose-level checks many times per day. Early in his life, he required a lot of supervision of his disease, and this demand pushed me even more to be an overly attentive father, perhaps even overprotective in an ultimately unhelpful way. These pressures on my wife and me caused us, and primarily me, to neglect our time together and created an eventually irreparable emotional distance.

In retrospect, I wonder if I could have been a better husband had I had a less-demanding career. Although my first marriage failed for many reasons, one big reason was that my training had emphasized there was no divorce allowed in my marriage to medicine.

My second marriage, in turn, was also short-lived and ended in divorce. Finally, by the time I gave marriage a third try, I felt more mature, and thus more able to balance the demands of medicine and marriage. I know that, now, I am a better partner.

My Military Service and Early Practice

After my child psychiatry fellowship, I became an "indentured servant" of the US Army. Like most physicians in the early 1970s, when the United States was at war in Vietnam, I entered medical school susceptible to the draft, but could, by choice, have my induction deferred until my training was complete. From the military's perspective, deferring a select group of physicians to allow them to complete their training in a specialty made sense, because they would eventually be more valuable in the armed services as specialists.

I underwent significant ethical conflict as a physician in the US Army. In the context of being the chief of psychiatry at an army hospital, I was instructed to perform psychiatric evaluations, but I knew that my patient records would not be privileged or confidential, as they would be available to nonmedical personnel. The individuals I examined had no rights—the needs of the military establishment came before theirs. I frequently found that the information I gathered about a patient could be detrimental to him. For example, if a soldier had a drug problem or was sexually involved with another enlisted person, such information could result in disciplinary action or even dishonorable discharge.

My personal method of dealing with this dilemma was to inform patients at the beginning of their sessions that my records were not confidential; that anything they told me could be used by the army in any manner seen fit; and that, as a physician, I could not protect their confidentiality.

There were a number of times when patients refused to talk to me, because whatever they needed to divulge could have a detrimental effect on their military career and thus the remainder of their lives. I felt that handling the ethical dilemma in this manner, however, was the best option. It was the most consistent with the oath I had taken to never do the patient harm.

Post-Military Practice

After serving three years in the military and treating a variety of cases, I decided upon a private practice back in Northern California, where I had gone to medical school. I was undecided as to whether I wanted an exclusively private practice, however, or a combination of academic medicine and private practice. So my first few years out of the army, I combined the two. On the academic side, I took a position at the University of California, San Francisco, as acting clinical director of the Center on Deafness, a mental-health facility serving the hearing-impaired.

This was a significant change for me in that I had had no experience working with deaf individuals and did not realize their unique psychiatric needs. The disability of deafness is not only one of not hearing, but also one in which you do not have the ability to effectively communicate; that is, you are not able to live in a society that is responsive to your needs or understanding of your unique language (sign language). The acquisition of language is what allows humans to modulate their own behavior, be less inclined to act out physically, and be more likely to talk about their frustrations and dysphoric feelings. Consequently, deaf people, without early language acquisition, may be more behaviorally disturbed, more impulsive, and more likely to act before reflecting.[7]

Working with the Deaf

Learning to work with this population was indeed a challenge. I learned sign language and primarily signed in what is called Signed Exact English, although I also became conversant with some deaf individuals in American Sign Language (ASL), the cultural language of the deaf. Learning to use Signed Exact English took several years of classes, and learning ASL was even more difficult, in that the sentence structure of the language is distinct from that in English. I don't believe I was ever close to being fluent in ASL.

At times, I needed to use an interpreter to help in my evaluation and treatment, but I found that I had a niche that made me unique, and, as a result, I quickly became an expert.

Initially, I certainly didn't consider myself an expert, but after twenty-plus years of experience, I now feel like I know the problems of deaf individuals relatively well. In that time, I have served as a consultant to the California School for the Deaf, seeing many patients in private practice, clinical settings, and hospitals. I have served as an expert witness in trials and given a number of lectures throughout the United States on the problems of deaf patients. For several years, in the early 1980s, I also helped evaluate candidates for the surgical procedure of cochlear implantation. At that time, cochlear implantation was considered a research project, but today, many deaf adults and children have had their functional hearing restored as a result of the procedure. I also ran a program at the University of California which attempted to facilitate the development of equal services for the hearing-impaired. It was a very difficult time, in that our program was unique and the demands it put on the clinicians working with me were significant. I consider myself lucky to have had an excellent staff of psychologists and social workers, however, and feel that we provided a great service while the program was thriving.

Moving into Full-Time Private Practice

In the early to mid-1980s, the picture changed somewhat. The State of California became less responsive to funding the specialized services we were promoting, and, as a result, the innovative programs we had established were starting to shrink. Moving away from a program that was novel in establishing satellite programs throughout various counties in Northern California, we found that we were unable to continue to grow and, instead, were forced to primarily serve deaf individuals in the immediate area of San Francisco. Struggling more and more with the administrative issues of the program and having less time for direct patient care, I decided to leave my academic position and move into full-time private practice.

While clinical director at the Center on Deafness, I had also maintained a part-time private practice and had found the rewards great. I was able to deliver good care, did not have any unusual difficulties with insurance companies, and maintained a flexible fee schedule, providing care for low-fee patients as well as regular-pay patients. Paperwork demands were considerable but not overwhelming.

Medi-Cal

One interesting sidelight of my full-time private practice was that, when I began, there was a Medi-Cal (state Medicaid) program in place. At that time, the standard psychotherapy fee was approximately sixty to eighty dollars per session. At that time, Medi-Cal paid about two-thirds of that fee, or forty dollars per individual patient session. That fee, although lower than what one would get from non-Medi-Cal patients, allowed the private practitioner enough of a payment that there was an incentive to serve indigent patients and those who were clearly in need of care but had no means to pay for it.

Now, almost thirty years later, while the fees for private care have at least doubled, the Medi-Cal rate for an individual psychotherapy session has increased by exactly one dollar, to forty-one dollars per session. Further, Medi-Cal is now run by each separate county in California. Because of that, I have been in the position of many psychiatrists in this state, having to severely curtail the number of Medi-Cal patients I see—another example of a failure of the state to provide for indigent people. Individual nonmedical clinicians provide most of the care of Medi-Cal patients. As a result, I now only see Medi-Cal patients at my job as a public psychiatrist at Sonoma County Community Mental Health, or in my job for a nonprofit agency contracted to provide mental-health services; I do not see them in my private practice.

The Problem with Paperwork

There has also been a tremendous increase in the paperwork demands and, at times, a sense that the state administrative structure not only has little regard for the delivery of service to Medi-Cal individuals, but also spends the majority of its time making it difficult for practitioners to provide them with necessary care. In the past year, as a service to several treatment facilities in my area, I have seen Medi-Cal recipients in emergencies and provided care. My secretary reported to me that the total amount charged for those services was approximately twenty-five hundred dollars, which she billed to Medi-Cal. After all of the red tape, returned claims, and bureaucratic lunacy or harassment we dealt with, however, I have been paid less than seven dollars for that twenty-five hundred dollars worth of care. My secretary put in approximately forty hours of clerical time on the claims.

I am not including this example to aggrandize my own image or good deeds, but to illustrate the pressure that all Californian physicians endure in trying to provide for medically indigent patients. Although Medi-Cal patients are now cared for under the counties' budgets, and not directly under the state's, the system remains abominable.

The Problem with Reviewers

One interesting sidelight to the inefficiency and stupidity of the entire Medi-Cal system is illustrated by the following story. When I began doing hospital work with Medi-Cal patients, I discovered that the person reviewing all of the psychiatric cases was not a psychiatrist. That person was an ophthalmologist, who seemed to have little knowledge of what was involved in psychiatric care. Denials of care were frequent, inexplicable, and seemingly based on some fiscal need of the state, as opposed to the clinical needs of the individuals.

I recall vividly that, on one occasion, this physician and I had a discussion on the telephone about the need for a patient to be in the hospital. Clearly, there was clinical indication of the person being depressed and in need of twenty-four-hour supervised care. Because of the thoroughness of my workup, I was able to pull out the fact that, on one occasion, the individual had used marijuana, but this fact only made the consultant feel that the patient had a substance-abuse problem, as opposed to depression. This tidbit about the patient in reference obviously did not make up the bulk of the evaluation; it was a minor part of the person's life history. But the ophthalmologist-consultant chose to focus on it, apparently as a method for denying the patient psychiatric care. His insensitivity insulted and outraged me, and led to a very heated discussion, which ended when I reminded him that both he and I had taken the same oath but that, clearly, he had forgotten his.

In the field of medicine, being trained in a particular specialty makes one "board-eligible." This eligibility allows the physician to take an exam administered by the appropriate medical board to become "board-certified." In my case, I took the exam and was certified by the American Board of Psychiatry and Neurology, with certification in general psychiatry and, several years later, in child and adolescent psychiatry. The government, however, often does not require the physicians reviewing cases for their various insurance programs, such as Medicaid and Medicare, to be board-certified. In other words, reviewing physicians are not required to have the adequate training or credentials to make judgments regarding the care that patients receive.

In the real, ethical world, however, recognition of the nature and depth of a physician's training is important. Only physicians with the proper training are qualified enough to make judgments about the treatment needs of patients with certain conditions. Mental-health patients need to be reviewed by psychiatrists—not surgeons or ophthalmologists.

Abuses within the System

During the mid-1970s to mid-1980s, the private practice I carried on in addition to my academic position brought me into contact with other doctors in my community. I believe I could say, without reservation, that 95 percent of those doctors, I respected. I felt they were knowledgeable and, without question, committed to their patients' care. I was impressed by the fact that there was a very high quality of medical care provided to the individuals in our community. However, I did recognize that, nationally, there were abuses within the system.

Unnecessary surgeries had, at times, been performed on patients, perhaps the most graphic being needless hysterectomies for relatively minor problems. Some doctors were rationalizing the need for certain types of care without closely monitoring what they were doing. There were doctors at weight-control clinics, for example, who used poor scientific methods, treating patients with questionable techniques and medications that seemed to dupe the insurance carriers, as well as the patients, out of money. And there were, as there are in any profession, certain individuals who would find loopholes in the system and abuse patients for their own gain. One example was the numerous surgeries being done on black infants for umbilical hernias, which any good physician knows is a condition that often clears with time and without surgical intervention. These practices were not going on in my community, but I had heard of them happening elsewhere.

For this reason—as a side note—if a patient is advised to have a procedure that seems unnecessary, he or she should request a second opinion from another physician who does not have a vested interest in either recommending or opposing the procedure. Second opinions are standard procedure in medicine, and, in my view, not utilized often enough. Insurance companies frequently feel second opinions are unnecessary expenses, without recognizing that it is the patient's right to be secure with a medical opinion, just as it is the insurance company's right to be fiscally sensible.

The Need for Monitoring

I also became aware during my early years of practicing that the field of medicine needed to monitor itself more closely. There needed to be utilization reviews, quality assurance, and peer reviews by doctors in outpatient practice. Any profession needs to ethically monitor itself to maintain standards. Although there were monitoring mechanisms in place, they were not adequate to handle the abuses that occurred, however infrequently. Medical leadership organizations were next to useless in controlling the profession, let alone in matching that control to the needs of society. For example, the American Medical Association and other specialty organizations like the American Psychiatric Association took, and continue to take, a reactive mode to medical crises rather than a proactive assessment of needs and trends, after which they might suggest innovative interventions.

Hippocrates tried to provide a code of behavior and ethics for a profession. The code is relatively straightforward and defined, but today's world and culture afford different pressures and challenges. Economic influences and new, extra-medical pressures manipulate the profession and obscure the ethical considerations. Physicians forget their areas of expertise, professional organizations poorly monitor, nonmedical professions assume medical competence, and the pressures on the practicing physician can result in poor patient care. The allegiance and focus of the physician need to be on the priority of good patient care, and other influences should not distract from that focus.

Corporate Medicine

When I went into full-time private practice, I wanted to combine that with more hospital work. Thus, I accepted a position as the medical director of a psychiatric unit in a private, for-profit, general medical hospital. One of my negotiating points for the position was that I could make this hospital unique by providing mental-health services for deaf people. As a part of my proposed program, the hospital would make interpreter services available so that deaf patients could be admitted and provided with quality care. The administrator of the psychiatric section of the hospital agreed to the idea, and so I began my work in this setting.

Gratifying Work

The first several years of that work were quite gratifying. The hospital census grew. Our average census when I began as medical director was about fifteen to twenty occupied beds; the peak census after one year was about forty occupied beds. We were able to establish an adolescent psychiatric unit and, later, a child psychiatric unit, and I believe the quality of care in both was generally quite high. Overall, I was blessed with an excellent staff, including good doctors as the admitting physicians in the hospital.

I did become aware of a trend, however, that was somewhat disturbing. Many psychiatrists gravitated toward outpatient practice exclusively and did very little inpatient work. Because of that, a certain percentage of the doctors who did inpatient work did so out of necessity, only because they could not establish an outpatient practice—and they probably could not establish an outpatient practice because the work they did was not well-received and their referrals not frequent enough to make the practice financially remunerative.

Problems with Inpatient Psychiatrists

This trend led to an interesting contradiction in the type of care required by inpatient clients and the quality of physicians providing for them. Inpatient work requires more time, attention, and availability by the physician, and also usually involves taking care of the more severely ill of the psychiatric population. Frequently, however, the least skilled psychiatrists were the ones doing the most hospital work, since these were the psychiatrists who could not make it exclusively in outpatient private practices. The selection process for doctors who primarily did inpatient work, then, had evolved into one in which, although they were less highly regarded in the community, they were available for referrals from crisis and hospital units who couldn't find any other doctors to take care of patients needing hospitalization.

Certainly, this trend didn't hold true for all of the inpatient psychiatrists, many of whom demonstrated great skill and superb patient care, but it did hold true for a significant percentage of inpatient psychiatrists that it seemed problematic to me.

Policing Treatment

One of my frustrations as medical director of the psychiatric portion of the general hospital was that I had to police the work of a number of physicians, and found that, at times, inadequate treatment was being administered—that is, treatment that had no rational basis in terms of the standard of care that should have been maintained. I had to tactfully learn to suggest more appropriate treatments to doctors, some of whom had been in practice for many more years than I had. Over time, I think I learned to do that relatively well.

Over time, I also became aware how crucial a hospital's nursing staff is in helping physicians who make questionable decisions to move in the right direction. A number of doctors at this hospital did not know their medications well, and did not understand the detrimental effects of using certain combinations of medications. It was only with the utmost tact and subtle redirection that nurses frequently helped these physicians to manage their patients in an acceptable manner.

Financial Aspects of Hospital Care

In the time I was medical director of this psychiatric unit, which had expanded into three units by the time I left—adult psychiatry, adolescent psychiatry, and child psychiatry—the financial pressures of hospital care seemed to increase exponentially. Psychiatric hospitals were springing up all over the country, and particularly all over Northern California, during this four- or five-year period in the early 1990s. Many units were being established because there had been a change in the California state law, which no longer required the demonstration of community need for hospitals. Consequently, an open competitive market existed. The emphasis of the hospital thus became one of marketing, which meant selling the hospital to the public in order to maintain a census adequate enough for the ownership of the company to make a profit.

Filling Beds

For me, marketing opened up a completely new arena of disillusionment in medical practice. Hospital administration began to listen to all sorts of wild claims by doctors who felt they could fill beds with unique, innovative programs, many of which had questionable virtue and capability. It is well documented throughout our country that, at this time, adolescents were frequently hospitalized in psychiatric facilities unnecessarily, purely because they had adequate insurance and because their families felt they needed to be in hospital settings, rather than because they actually had psychiatric illnesses requiring such a setting.

The best example would be those kids who, because they had bad grades or some sort of conduct problem, were hospitalized rather than given adequate learning experiences or placed in juvenile detention centers, both of which would be more appropriate solutions to help them deal with their issues. Often, adolescents who'd had normal teenage conflicts with their parents were placed in hospitals, given wastebasket diagnoses such as "adjustment disorder" or "adolescent turmoil," and then discharged when they abruptly began to suffer from what I call "insurance deficiency syndrome," meaning their insurance coverage had been exhausted.

A number of years ago, a television program such as *20/20* or *60 Minutes* ran a feature story and gave many examples of these kinds of exploitative hospitals and their marketing practices. Fortunately, the hospital I worked with did not seem to be in that kind of bind.

It was, however, in the bind of a decreasing census, because of the bourgeoning of psychiatric beds throughout the Northern California area.

New Company, Different Philosophy

Several years after I became the medical director of the psychiatric unit at this private hospital, the larger hospital, which was owned by Republic Corporation, closed. Since the psychiatric unit had been a portion of the private hospital, which was making money, it remained open as a freestanding psychiatric facility.

With the closing of the larger hospital, however, a number of very interesting alterations occurred. The first was that the parent company that owned the private hospital declared Chapter 11. With this change in financial viability, the psychiatric unit was transferred to another parent company, which came in with a very different philosophy and certainly more aggressive tactics for managing staffing patterns and the quality of patient care.

I had a great deal of difficulty, often struggling with the administration over the quality of medical care. It was clear to me that nursing staff were frequently being let go and that inadequate nursing was being maintained purely for fiscal reasons, without concern for the maintenance of patient safety and care. Since then, as I have reflected on other such freestanding psychiatric hospitals, I have come to see them as parasitic, exploiting psychiatric patients and the tremendous gap that exists in monitoring these patients' care. Because these patients frequently are not able to protect themselves as much as other patient groups might be, they are more vulnerable to abuses.

One attraction when I started at the private psychiatric hospital was the good feeling I had about the administrator who ran the program. When the hospital became a freestanding psychiatric hospital, I began to notice that he was under tremendous pressure from the new parent owners to cut costs and increase patient census. He would spend extreme amounts of time on the phone with the vice president of the parent company, which was located in Texas, even though we were in Northern California. There were at least daily phone calls to him questioning the census, and he seemed to be under constant criticism if the census dipped even for a day. He was no longer given free rein to develop programs, and, in his reports to me, began to exceedingly highlight the business aspects of medical care.

Horizon Mental Health Corporation

After a period of time in this intense situation, the administrator resigned and returned to the private practice of psychology. With his departure, the parent company, Horizon Mental Health Corporation, brought in a new administrator, and my disillusionment increased tremendously.

As a sideline, it was always intriguing to me that, when I took my job as medical director of the psychiatric unit, the general hospital was owned by the Republic Corporation. As I mentioned before, the Republic Corporation experienced financial setbacks and filed for bankruptcy. However, the psychiatric portion of the hospital was still sold, or somehow transferred, to a mental-health group called Horizon Mental Health Corporation. Thus, upon very short notice, and with very little publicity, we became one of Horizon Mental Health Corporation's freestanding psychiatric units. I had always wondered how this process had occurred, and later, when further abuses of the mental-health system became publicized, wondered even more.

I then noticed that, in the book *The Great White Lie,* by Walt Bogdanich, the Republic Health Corporation is mentioned as one of the companies with questionable business practices during this time.[8] I am in no way implying that I had knowledge of anything illegal going on, but I have always questioned how this kind of transaction could occur.

Wooing Doctors

In any case, the move to ownership under the Horizon Corporation was a true eye-opener for me. The administrator they selected, from my vantage point, was an abomination. He started his position with a great deal of energy, requesting multiple meetings with doctors in the community, with a heavy emphasis on wooing them to hospitalize their patients with us. He talked about having a car wash for the doctors, so they could bring their cars in and get them washed by hospital staff. He would deliver birthday baskets to their offices in person or via one of his staff members. He put excessive energy into marketing the hospital and finding new venues for luring patients into our care.

A number of incidents that arose from his efforts were exceedingly appalling. For example, when he purchased season tickets for the San Francisco 49ers for use by the medical staff. The tickets were obviously quite costly, and his techniques were gauche at best; on one occasion, he had several doctors transported to a 49ers game in a limousine.

Another appalling incident was a discussion he had with a group of psychiatrists in San Francisco, in which he invited their patients to our hospital and suggested he would provide for their transportation—in fact, limousine transportation, if they so desired. What was becoming of medical care? Where had quality landed on this new priority list? Rarely were the words "quality of patient care" a focus of the new administration's concern.

I and other members of the medical staff who were offended by this administrator's actions raised these issues. As medical director, I had several weekly meetings with the unit directors and the offending hospital director. I also had many individual meetings with the hospital director during which I expressed my concern about the focus on profit rather than quality care. Most of the disillusioned medical staff expressed their opinions privately, in one-to-one conversations with me. The unit chiefs, three other physicians, were not very vocal about their concerns. And as time went on, I became more and more disenchanted with his techniques and unsure whether they were really supported by Horizon Corporation.

What if Horizon did support him? I was appalled, at times, to hear the comptroller of our hospital talk about how easy it was to deceive insurance carriers and especially government carriers (e.g.,

Medicare) about what services were being provided for patients, and to hear that standard practice in the hospital's business office, at times, was to "pad bills," attaching expenditures to patient bills that were of questionable or totally fraudulent validity.

I also vividly remember a medical staff meeting with a dinner menu that would have made any quality San Francisco restaurant proud: beef Wellington, prawns, oysters, elaborate desserts, champagne, wine, and so on. I was struck with the fact that the cost had obviously been very great, with fifty to one hundred doctors present, but that two social workers had just been told the hospital could not afford to keep them on staff. Cuts had also been planned for the creative art staff. Why the contradiction? Why did Horizon provide such excesses, yet have so little regard for quality medical care that they felt justified in drastically cutting the heart of the program? I could not understand.

Voicing My Concerns for Quality Care

It was this situation, and others like it, which eventually prompted me to ask for a meeting with the vice president of Horizon Corporation. He and his assistant came to Marin County, and I took him to lunch—probably one of the rare occasions when a doctor spent money on Horizon Corporation versus the other way around. I talked about my concerns with the direction of the hospital, the apparent apathy regarding the quality of patient care, and the marketing techniques being used by the administrator.

His response was very noncommittal. He was clearly business-oriented in his approach, using all the right words, but there was something about him I did not trust. In fact, there was something about him that I found outright despicable.

About two weeks after that discussion, he announced that he and his assistant would be doing an evaluation of the hospital programs and leadership, and would come up with recommendations for improvement. Those recommendations, as it turned out, were quite interesting. Within a day after the evaluations, the administrator was dismissed from his position, a move that was met with great relief by the staff. That relief was quickly shattered, however, when, at the same time, we learned that I had been asked to resign as medical director. It is interesting that I was asked to resign; I was not fired. I could not have been fired unless I had been remiss in carrying out my duties.

Instead, I was told by the vice president of Horizon Corporation that my philosophy did not mesh with theirs, and, although he had the "utmost respect" for me "as a person and as a psychiatrist providing quality care," he did not feel that, philosophically, I should continue as medical director. His statement, again, was interesting, since the Horizon Corporation never had a mission statement for the hospital or a philosophical statement about their approach to medical care.

In retrospect, I surmised that the administrator had been acting under the sanction of Horizon Mental Health, who probably realized that, if they kept me in the position of medical director, any new administrator they put in that position would have difficulty. After all, I wouldn't ethically allow the things that had been going on to continue without "raising a ruckus."

For a time, I did not resign, even though they had wanted me to within two weeks. I reminded them that I had a contract, which, unless they could point out to me something I'd been doing wrong, was still in force. I told them that I would certainly be willing to leave the position, however, if they bought out the remainder of my contract period. Suddenly, they seemed to achieve clarity regarding the fact that they had no grounds for dismissing me and that doing so would cost them money, and they backed off from their position. The whole process had, however, also opened my eyes to the reality that I would have to leave the position, regardless of the contract. Very shortly thereafter, I gave them notice that I would be terminating, probably to their relief. I stopped being medical director in late 1992.

Support from My Staff

Most heartening to me, and something that I will forever appreciate, is that, when I was asked to leave as medical director, there was almost uniformity among the staff in the opinion that that move should not occur. There were well over a hundred signatures on a petition asking for clarification from the parent company as to why the change would occur.

Since we were dealing with a private enterprise system, neither the outcry from the medical staff nor that from the hospital employees altered their stance that my philosophy "was not compatible" with theirs. What was apparent to the staff, however, was that my philosophy was one in which patient care, quality care, and ethical care should come first, which left little room for interpretation about the philosophy of the parent company, given that they'd stated their position was contrary to mine.

Meeting with the FBI

An interesting sideline to this story was that, shortly after I left the position of medical director, I discovered that the assistant to the vice president was under investigation and perhaps indictment in Texas. The accusation against him was in regard to fraud at a hospital that he'd headed in the Denton, Texas, area. The information had been printed in the professional monthly publication, the *Psychiatric Times*.[9]

It is also of interest that, on two occasions after I left the hospital, the FBI requested confidential meetings with me, in which they came to my office and questioned me extensively about the dealings of the hospital and the Horizon Corporation. I was a little apprehensive about the meetings, even though the interviews involved answering questions not about my personal practices or myself, but only about what I knew of the hospital's practices. The FBI agent who met with me was quite personable and seemed genuinely interested in finding out facts and pursuing issues. As far as the intricacies of the ethical dealings of the corporation and the hospital, however, I had virtually no information for him. I told him I was involved only in the hospital's medical operations. Apart from saying that I didn't like what I gleaned as the "greed orientation" and lack of human compassion of some of the corporate officers, I don't think I provided much help for the FBI inquiry. I was informed that the FBI did not want me to discuss these issues with the newspapers, however, as it might raise problems in their investigation.

The interviews occurred in late 1992 or early 1993, and were not something I'd gone through before, and have never gone through since. To date, I do not know the outcome of the FBI investigation or even whether any progress was made. It did happen, however, that some time after they questioned me, the comptroller of the hospital left his job, and, again, the ownership changed. It was transferred to a company called the Orynda Corporation. A new hospital administrator told me that Orynda Corporation is still owned in part by the same individuals who owned Horizon Corporation.

Again, all of the intricacies of these business dealings are unknown to me. Whether they were standard practice or questionable is unclear; neither is it necessarily to be construed that anything illegal occurred. Whenever such business situations heat up, patterns of transfer cast some suspicion over the way business changes occur.

Parasites

My resignation as the hospital's medical director actually came as a relief to me. I had freed myself from the burden of working for a parasitic group that seemed to prey on mental-health patients, and felt, perhaps, I could go back to seeing patients in the office—working in a situation in which I could provide quality care under my control, and not under the control of business interests.

How naïve I had been to think that, since the period of managed care was only just starting to rear its ugly head. Little did I know that the intrusion of business into medicine was only gradually coming into focus and that more parasites were to come.

What are parasites? In nature, parasites are biological beings that latch onto hosts and survive off of them. Unappreciative of their host life form, they take what they need, not contributing any good to the host, but, instead, creating illness in it. Indeed, if the host dies, they move on, trying to find another.

Corporate hospitals and most HMOs are the parasites of medical care. Their goal is high profit, at all costs. If the field of medicine becomes ill as a result, they do not notice. If they ruin or kill quality care, they do not care, as long as the profit margin is high. Some of them recognize that their life span will be relatively short, so they take as much profit as they can—and to hell with suffering or death.

Particularly in psychiatry, corporate parasites now run rampant. They move in on a relatively helpless patient group and corrupt doctors with promises of quality and money, never with the intent to provide quality and providing money only so long as the profit margin is great. In places where quality exists at first, as the profit bundle begins to fall below a certain point, that quality becomes expendable. Greed runs rampant and the intent is to rape and pillage until discovered, and then to move onto new, untouched territory. Meanwhile, patients suffer, lives are lost, and eventually the host just dies.

My experience at the hospital began with great promise. I was the pawn. I started the adolescent service, the children's service, and the deaf program. We had national exposure, high census, and high profit. Then the greed took over, and I challenged the ethics, irritating the parasite. I dared to expose the greed, and I kept focusing on quality.

Look at the deaf program; it's expensive and brings in only a modest return on the money. So, skew the statistics (as Mark Twain said, "there are lies, damn lies, and statistics") and say it's losing money. Then, as a solution, start shrinking the number of child and adolescent beds. Combine the adolescent unit with the chemical-dependency unit. As bizarre and unbelievable as this solution seems, that is what actually happened. Slowly most programs were compromised, and the hospital's demise loomed. And do not tell the outside community about any of the changes and compromised patient care. The parasite continues to eat right up until the host ultimately dies.

Providing Quality Care

During my entire time at the hospital, I continued to be impressed with my colleagues. For the most part the doctors I worked with were of excellent quality. If anything, they were bewildered by the business aspects of medicine—naïve babes in the woods. What I respected and continue to respect most about them was that, despite all that was happening around them, they were still able to provide quality medical care, treating the patients well.

Even now, of all the doctors I know in my community who are practicing medicine of any kind, I believe that 95 percent or more are exceedingly ethical, dedicated, quality individuals whose patients' best interests is their motivation for continuing their practice.

I do, however, hear their disillusionment, often in statements that begin with, "If I had to choose whether to go into medicine again or not … " And approximately 50 percent of them say they wouldn't. In fact, when the children of these physicians ask about going into medicine, many of the doctors tell them not to, for the sole reason that medicine is so different today than when they began practicing.

Ethical Dilemmas

The patient-centered Hippocratic tradition has become more of an ethical dilemma to today's practitioners. Confidentiality has perhaps become the most prevalent type of ethically troubling incident for the mental-health professional. Patients' medical histories, collected by insurance companies, are placed on computers with nationwide networks to document preexisting conditions. Patient records documenting psychiatric conditions, which still have a stigma attached to them in today's society, are made available to individuals who work for the insurance industry without these workers' oath of confidentiality or the patients' knowledge. Insurance companies also, at times, ask for detailed notes from the psychiatrist about the nature of patients' conflicts.

As the exact content of a patient's interview should be protected, I will never release verbatim notes of what my patients discuss in their sessions. I will only provide a psychiatric assessment and discussion of their symptoms with a patient's permission. I made the decision to not share specific notes—except with trained medical personnel or, if ordered, with the court—with one of the first patients I saw in private practice. She was an adolescent of about age seventeen who was depressed and talked at length about her controlling father. She was in treatment for around six months, and her condition improved. During this time, I had periodic meetings with her parents to inform them of her progress. After she terminated her treatment, I had a request from her attorney father for all of my files on his daughter, including all of my written notes. Since releasing that material would involve divulging her personal negative feelings about the controlling nature of her father, along with other destructive feelings toward other family members, I felt I could not do that. It would betray her trust and potentially harm her. The father demanded the notes, however, and stated he would not pay her last bill until he received the file. I explained that his daughter's emotional well-being was more important than the money, and told him that if he could disregard his daughter's feelings over a few hundred dollars, I chose not to collaborate. I never collected on the final bill, and the father didn't receive the file.

Another ethical dilemma that has arisen: some physicians argue that the patient focus required by the Hippocratic Oath is in conflict with forensic medicine, and that frequently, in both contested and noncontested situations, patients are examined not for the benefit of the patient but for the benefit of the legal process.

In the past, physicians had a traditional focus on the Hippocratic Oath; that is, only as it applied to the doctor-patient relationship. As society has become more complex, however, so has the physician's role in that relationship. It has always been good medical practice, in problematic diagnostic situations, to have a second or third medical opinion, but if that opinion is provided by a doctor with a vested interest in pleasing the payer of his or her fee, (e.g., the insurance company or lawyer), there's a higher risk that the opinion, consciously or unconsciously, might be slanted to suit the physician's best financial position.

Now apply this idea to physicians who do a lot of legal work, for example, those who are frequently hired to examine patients as expert witnesses. If a law firm is footing the bill for that doctor's time, and the doctor produces a diagnosis or conclusion contrary to what the referring lawyer is seeking, it is unlikely that physician will receive future referrals from that law firm.

That's why, whenever a physician testifies in a legal case, he or she is frequently asked the question, "How many times have you testified for the defense and how many times for the plaintiff?" The point of the question is that, if the physician's testimony is slanted too far in one direction, the doctor is likely just a "hired gun" whose opinion is for sale. Another question commonly asked of testifying physicians is, "Are you being paid for your medical opinion?" The correct answer is, "No, I'm being paid for my time. My opinion is determined by the patient's condition." But the point of the question is the same.

Another ethical dilemma has occurred over the last two decades as a result of the increased emphasis on patient autonomy and informed consent, which has significantly changed both physician and patient values. Traditionally, the doctor-as-patient-advocate received the broadest attention, and, as such, the physician's focus was predominantly on both doing the best for the individual patient as well as on doing no harm. Today, as opposed to this "doctor knows best" value system, the patient has at least as much say in choosing or refusing treatment as the physician does.

In addition, in some instances in today's society, the definition of "patient" is now being broadened to include groups of patients. Thus, in certain systems, the physician may need to advocate for a group of patients rather than an individual. Groups, however, may choose systems of care that ration, allocate, capitulate, or in some other manner divide resources among a whole group. Individuals who prescribe to a group insurance plan are usually not aware of the implications of doing so, or may have had the plan chosen for them by their employers or insurance agents.

In the public sector, rationing or allocation plans are currently being implemented as well. In care to the medically indigent, for example, Medicaid has very restrictive practices for coverage, and the needs of the group usually take precedence over the needs of the individual.

Individuals under these groups, both private and public, are often not informed of the subjugation of the need of the individual to the need of the group when it comes to their health care. It affects the very fabric of our nation, and yet the individuals subject to it have had it imposed upon them without their knowledge or consent, often only becoming aware of the limitations during a state of illness. Many may argue that people should know what their policies cover by reading them, but the reality is that, frequently, policies are not read until an illness occurs, and insuring companies do not make their clients aware of any policy limitations until the clients ask them pointed questions leading to such information. Such questions usually only arise at the time of a client's illness, and the result is compromised care.

Another example of insurance clients being kept in the dark: when patients sign up for medical coverage under one particular insurance group, they must sign that they will not file malpractice suits but rather, on all contested issues, agree to arbitration. An arbitrated case is much more likely to result in a lower award to the offended patient, but most of these people do not realize that they signed an arbitration agreement because they have not read their policies.

Insurance's Invasion into the Practice of Medicine

As a private practitioner, I have frequently had to deal with health insurance companies. I have recently found that several insurance companies insist patients in need of mental-health services see a marriage, family, and child counselor (MFCC) before seeing a psychiatrist, principally because the MFCC costs less. These insurance companies also insist that the MFCC put down a medical diagnosis for the patient, despite the fact that—at least within California—MFCCs are not qualified to make medical diagnoses; they are only qualified to deal with relationship conflicts.

Practicing Medicine without a License
In essence, the insurance companies and managed health-care providers in such cases are encouraging the practicing of medicine without a license. This could not be to the patient's benefit, and I have seen a number of patients as proof that it is not. Many patients who come to me, who have seen MFCCs first, have been previously misdiagnosed or incorrectly delayed treatment as a result.

Over the years, practitioners from other disciplines, for example, psychologists, social workers, and others, have joined the process of aiding people with problems that involve the mind. Many of these practitioners erroneously call their patient assessments "psychiatric evaluations." Meanwhile, the general public is usually unaware that, out of all the practitioners of mental-health disciplines, psychiatrists are the only ones qualified with the medical training to perform such evaluations. Therefore, the incorrect labeling of such evaluations continues unchallenged.

In addition, the problem could worsen, as many clinical psychologists are trying to lobby for the right to prescribe medication without attending medical school. These psychologists are proposing they receive only a miniscule amount of training in pharmacology. God help us if they're successful.

There are 954,000 physicians in the United States whose medical training included studies in human anatomy, physiology, microbiology, pathology, biochemistry, and other multiple specialties. Yet many health-care professionals with much less training seem to feel they have expertise that is equal, or at least similar, to that of a physician. Nurse practitioners, physicians' assistants, optometrists, nurse anesthetists, and a wide range of other health-care practitioners, for example, are increasingly expressing the wish to become more autonomous—and separate from medicine.

The discipline of psychiatry is no exception to this rule. Psychiatrists are continually faced with practitioners of other professional disciplines who have little to no medical training trying to perform their medical role. Counselors, social workers, pastors, nurse practitioners, "addictionologists," and "rent-a-friends" all seem to, at times, confuse their disciplines with that of psychiatry.

I believe my training helped me understand the wide implication of the human condition. It also qualified me to properly treat and prescribe medication to patients. And given the magnitude of such a responsibility, I do not believe there is a shortcut to that type of expertise.

Saving Money

I once discussed the idea that other professions were increasingly impinging upon the psychiatrist's role as physician with one of the vice presidents of a health maintenance organization—a psychiatrist, no less. He seemed surprised that I had an objection to it and could only state that the practice probably needed to continue because of financial reasons. I hardly found that an acceptable explanation. After all, mental health may be the portent of what is to come for the rest of medicine. I can imagine that, carried to the extreme, the next step would be for insurance companies to insist that all patients be seen first by a nurse practitioner, who would diagnose the patient before he or she is referred to the appropriate specialist or even to a primary care doctor. This would be in the service of saving money, but certainly not in the patients' best medical interest.

The amount of money the insurance industry makes is phenomenal. My position, after trying to deal with this industry for many years now, is that it is motivated purely for profit and that it prescribes to no code of ethics or oath that dictates that patients' needs come first. Therefore, it's time for that industry to be removed from the doctor-patient relationship.

Medicine's Contribution to the Mess

It's clear that medicine has helped create its own problem. Over the years, there's been a well-publicized litany of fraud and waste. Take the following situations, for example:

- Unnecessary uses of technology, for example, a relatively small community having multiple magnetic resonance scanners, when one shared scanner would be more reasonable and lower the overall cost of procedures.
- Communities establishing more hospital beds than needed.
- Physicians owning their own laboratories or pharmacies and having vested interests in ordering more tests or more expensive medications than necessary.
- Doctors performing unnecessary procedures when they are not clinically indicated.
- Doctors and hospitals "unbundling" procedures to make more money.

Unbundling

Unbundling is a process whereby the billing of a medical procedure is done by breaking the procedure into its component parts and charging for each part individually, rather than charging a standard or more reasonable cost for the total procedure. An example might be billing for a routine oophorectomy/hysterectomy by charging for the removal of the ovaries separately from the removal of the uterus, and—if the first operation on the patient's abdomen—also issuing a separate charge for the standard removal of the appendix. The bills for all of these procedures together amounts to a total charge far in excess of the usual cost of the procedure, and the resulting cost to the insurance company or patient becomes exorbitant.

Using an experience from my own life, I now know that there was unbundling going on at the psychiatric hospital while I was the medical director there. It worked something like this: The standard fee for a patient's stay in the hospital was X amount of dollars. As insurance companies became increasingly restrictive on patients using the hospital, however, the hospital began to negotiate separate rates with separate insurance companies. They also began unbundling hospital charges. Before unbundling, the total price for one day included nursing care, group therapy, social work services, occupational therapy, art therapy, movement therapy, and so one. After unbundling, the basic rate included only the patient's room and board, and every service beyond that, if possible, was billed separately. There would be Charge X for room and board, plus Charge Y for group therapy, plus Charge Z for social work, and on and on the charges went for as many services as could be unbundled. The return for the hospital was enormous.

Other Abuses

Pharmaceutical companies have patents on medications that last for years and years, and elevate the cost. The cost dramatically drops, however, as soon as the patent runs out and there are competing companies on the market. It is my sense that these patents exist for far too long and that reform is needed in this area.

Another area with significant problems is in worker compensation claims. Doctors have made excessive amounts of money dealing with these claims, frequently generating lengthy reports for which they can charge substantial fees, despite such reports being largely computer-generated and including a great deal of useless information. I know of doctors who, despite the fact that the computer has done the majority of the billable time on a report, will bill for hours and hours of work on it.

In the past, there were few restrictions on creating such large bills, and workers' compensation medicine was a very lucrative practice, with a number of physicians establishing "mills," hiring other doctors to do the workups for patients and becoming quite wealthy as a result. However, relatively recently, at least in the state of California, this practice has come under investigation and a ceiling has been put in place to limit the costs.

Perhaps the severity and far-reaching effects of such abuses can be best demonstrated by an article I read years ago. It appeared in the August 1999 issue of *Psychiatric Times*, a monthly newspaper distributed to psychiatrists. The article stated that a psychiatrist who treated one of the Menendez brothers later openly admitted that, as a result of his discussions with the defense counsel, changed some of his records and notes. He changed them in the course of the trial, and he changed them for the sole purpose of presenting a better picture of his former patient. More unbelievable is that this psychiatrist, at least in the article, expressed no recognition of the damage he had done to the profession; he seemed to demonstrate a complete lack of ethical perspective. He also failed to acknowledge that he had made a horrible error and that what he had done was a crime.

No one questions the fact that abuses have occurred and that poor monitoring within the medical profession has failed to eliminate these abuses. (This is why monitoring must occur in any plan set up in the future.) However, because of the ethical pledges of physicians to care for patients, the bottom line is that the patient-doctor relationship remains intact. Unfortunately, under the present system, even that cannot exist very often. Neither would it exist under some of the proposed plans. For example, many patients I've seen have been disenchanted by the fact that they have been denied access to their primary care physicians because of the insurance they carry. Further, in some instances, unless a physician agrees to operate under the business guidelines proposed by a particular insurance company, a patient cannot see that doctor. Those business guidelines, however, may involve a subtle requirement to compromise care and to enable the insurance or managed care company to dictate the needs of the patient, while keeping the physician liable for the outcome. Finally, there seems to be an epidemic of fraud in the medical industry, by a few individuals and by a great number of managed care companies.

Managed care, then, from my perspective, has been mangled care.

Insecurity about Health Care

I believe that, within the United States, there is a universal insecurity about medical-care coverage. Businesses that spend large amounts of money on insurance benefits for their employees are suffering, and massive numbers of individuals in this country are suffering more. The medically indigent population is growing, and millions of individuals without any medical insurance are being denied access to quality care. For most of the elderly or Social-Security-qualified disabled individuals, trying to deal with the bureaucracy of Medicare is exceedingly difficult. And anyone who develops a chronic illness faces great challenges getting any medical attention whatsoever. In fact, some insurance companies exclude these latter patients as soon as the chronic condition is diagnosed.

I recently had occasion to be referred by a managed care organization, which asked me to do a psychiatric consultation on a patient. I saw the patient, a child, four times, and sent the insurance a report, which included a diagnosis of a condition they considered chronic. They denied payment for the referral, and then sent the patient's family and me letters saying that the patient would be responsible for payment of my services, because a chronic condition had been found. How could that be? How could a managed care company opt out of paying for a consultation just because the outcome of that consultation had been a diagnosis of a chronic condition? Trying to deal with the physician-owner of that managed care company led to no satisfaction on my part—only disdain and disgust for him and his practices. Obviously, he was a doctor who had abandoned his Hippocratic Oath, lost his ability to see patients' needs, and opted to prioritize the business end of medical practice over good patient care.

The medical industry is now an industry in turmoil, creating great panic for both doctors and patients. It almost appears that this society is punishing sick people rather than treating them.

As you look at other countries, many are further along than the United States in dealing with this health-care crisis. In this country, as early as President Harry Truman's administration, there was a discussion about the need for national health insurance. It came up at other times, as well, but blossomed during the Clinton administration, and, for a time, appeared as if the issue would finally be addressed by President Obama. Now, however, it appears to have been consumed by inertia and is a political bomb that neither of the two main parties has the guts to tackle. Whenever health-care reform is discussed, the idea seems to be embraced by the public, but if and when and how such reform might take place is currently a mystery.

Health Care in Other Countries

Other countries have handled medical care in different ways. A great debate exists over whether Canada has an acceptable system or not.

Journalist Rhonda Hackett published an article in the *Denver Post* on June 7, 2009, that summarizes her experience with the Canadian system and compares it favorably with the US system.[10] There are negative myths that need to be exposed about abuses and cost of the care in the Canadian Health Plan. Why these myths are generated I do not know, but I am sure the United States insurance companies in favor of the status quo do nothing to dispel the false information.

Japan's program seems to cover costs from cradle to grave but has absolutely no frills and is clearly—or so it appears to me on close scrutiny—a system inferior to one the United States would want. Newspaper reporter Blaine Harden, writing in the *Washington Post* on September 7, 2009, summarized the Japanese system and concluded the cost may not be sustainable.[11]

Germany also has nationalized health insurance but seems bent on curbing costs with great pressure on patients and physicians; many people there have been denied care because of arbitrary decisions and long, unnecessary waits. Princeton University Economics Professor Uwe E. Reinhardt, in the publication *Economix* on April 17, 2009, in an article entitled "Health Reform without a Public Plan: The German Model" critiques the models of the Netherlands, Switzerland, and Germany and concludes that the real question is whether "America's private health insurers would be willing to countenance the tight regulation required for that approach."[12]

Domestic Health Care

Within this country, a number of states have attempted to set up their own programs. Hawaii has a system in place, and Oregon uses a program of social triage. The state of New York has several programs being touted as pilot projects, particularly managed care programs for Medicaid patients.

The dilemma I have as a physician is that I do not understand all of the economics involved in delivery of proper care. What I do see from a doctor's perspective, however, is insurance fraud, suffering patients, and the need for a significantly different system than what currently exists.

President Clinton did not respond to these needs and opted for the status quo, perpetuating the existing dysfunctional system. The most recent Republican administration did not look for a solution and succumbed to pressure from the insurance industry to maintain what was already there.

In 2008 and 2009 in California, there was a movement for a single-payer system modeled after the Canadian system. This movement failed after the opposition, funded primarily by the insurance industry, spent an estimated six to seven times the amount of money in defeating it as was spent by proponents. This system would have eliminated individual companies as insurers of medical care and put in their place a program that would provide medical care for all and the option for individual patients to select the physicians of their choice.

Removing competing, profit-motivated health insurance companies from the system is only one part of the solution to the problem, however. The only real solution would be a revolution in health-care needs, with several key guidelines and inviolate covenants, which we will get to more in last chapter of the book. A revamping of the total system is absolutely necessary.

Brain Drain

If the current system continues or an improper new system is established, there is a great danger of "brain drain" in the industry—that is, medicine runs the risk of losing competent physicians in their prime, due to excessive frustration that ultimately leads to burnout. Said more simply, good physicians will leave the practice due to their increasing frustrations with the medical bureaucracy.

I am already aware of some older, financially secure doctors who have retired early due to the fact that a proper system has not been established. Other older doctors are threatening to retire early, should they receive any more pressure that interferes with their capability to put the patients' needs first and to practice the kind of medicine they have been trained to practice. The intrusion into the quality of patient care is simply too great an ethical dilemma for these men and women.

I believe this dilemma exists for some younger and middle-aged physicians, as well, who are finding alternatives to private practice or switching to new careers that remove them from the ethical conundrums created by the current direction of medicine.

As a result of this brain drain, in my California county, more than half of the primary care physicians are leaving the practice in the next five years, and very few new physicians are coming into the state.[13] Conversely, I know of many doctors who, if the ethical frustrations of medicine lessened, would continue to practice for many, many years, even beyond retirement, as long as they were intellectually capable of doing so.

I believe this is a tragedy. It takes a long time to become a compassionate, concerned physician, and if we drive our older and better doctors out of medicine, then we, as a country, are going to lose.

Managed Competition

In the early 1980s, a large group of insurance carriers called health maintenance organizations (HMOs) began to invade the health-care industry with a new form of insurance delivery. Besides HMOs, there were also PPOs (preferred provider organizations), IPAs (independent practitioner associations or independent physicians associations), and multiple other entities with mystifying abbreviations. Doctors were inundated with a variety of alphabetized acronyms, which proved confusing to patients and medical professionals alike.

A Dramatic Change in Health-Care Delivery

Along with these new carriers came literally hundreds of contracts for doctors to sign in order to become a part of the various organizations. The predominant thinking was that it behooved the physician to sign up for these programs, so that they would be able to continue to provide care for whoever walked through the door.

Since most physicians, including me, have very little business sense, we failed to realize that this was the beginning of a dramatic change in health-care delivery. The responsibility for the payment of care was shifting from the patient to the insurance carrier, with the patient having responsibility only for the copayment, and the contracting physician being required to accept whatever fee was stated in the contract. And too frequently, billing statements were obscure and misleading.

For example, under the Blue Cross system in Northern California, the physician's customary charge for individual psychotherapy was listed at one hundred fifteen dollars, a fee acceptable to most psychiatrists. In actuality, the patient was covered for only twenty dollars of that visit. That meant the patient's portion was ninety-five dollars. Complicating the picture was the fact that Blue Cross also had a contract for the delivery of services under Medicare. The physician provider, then, might be limited in the amount that he or she could bill for the services covered by the Medicare portion of the contract—roughly seventy-five dollars, if you were a participating physician. The patient would be responsible for half of that, and Medicare would pay the other half. Therefore, instead of the reasonable and customary rates, suddenly the doctor was collecting less than 80 percent of the usual fee. Compounding that problem was the fact that a substantial amount of time had to be invested in filling out forms and billing these programs.

Returning, Losing, and Kiting Claims

Very few physicians had time to see patients and keep up with the paperwork. Each insurance entity had a different form and different requirements. One entity, in particular, required a fifteen-page form to be filled out for my services. That paperwork requirement lasted only a short time, however, as the HMO went out of business. Granted, this particular instance was peculiar to psychiatry, but the implications were, and still are, there for all aspects of medicine.

Further, upon investigation, many HMOs stated that it did not matter how correctly the billing forms were completed and submitted, as 50 percent of them would be returned. Many years ago, I was treating a patient who worked for one of the major insurance deliverers. She said that her supervisor informally told her that a sizable percentage of the company's forms should be "lost." Their reasoning for this was that, since patients and physicians alike frequently gave up on the collection of approximately half of the claims filed, whatever that uncollected money amounted to would be pure profit for the carrier. Returning 50 percent of the forms to their originating medical providers, regardless of how correctly they'd been filled out, also kept money in the insurance company's pocket until the claim was resubmitted, perhaps for a second, third, or fourth time, and the carriers were finally forced to pay up.

Meanwhile, these carriers paid very little attention to calls from physicians' offices. They gave much more attention to calls from patients who were irate that their medical bills were not being paid, however.

There were other times when it was clear that insurance companies were taking excessive time to cover medical bills. In the wider world, this is called "kiting." Because of this phenomenon, laws were passed to limit the amount of time insurance carriers were allowed to withhold payment. Now, if that time limit is exceeded, patients may complain to the Insurance Commissioner's Office in California.

Shrinking Profit Margins for Physicians

After the entrance of the HMO, the physician came to be seen as the enemy, an individual with a vested interest in taking money from the insurance company. Most physicians, however, were paying little attention to the fact that their usual and customary fees were being whittled down to a small percentage of what they had been. Add this to the fact that most physicians' offices had to expand their ancillary personnel staff at considerable costs just to keep up with this tremendous demand in paperwork, and the profit margin for seeing patients was reduced even further.

Interestingly enough, in my own practice, I recently calculated that if I paid to bring in an expert to look at the management of my company at the usual fee for one year—a rate of forty dollars per hour for a forty-hour week—he or she would make more money than I would. And I'm a well-respected psychiatrist in my community, with more patients than I can possibly see requesting my services. What about a physician just starting out, trying to build a practice? Had I more business savvy, I would have recognized this trend far before it had gotten out of hand. However, like most physicians, I get far more gratification from dealing with patients than with paperwork or insurance companies. So when HMOs entered the scene, the business aspects of my practice took a back seat to my Hippocratic Oath and the wish to deliver the best service possible to my patients.

Interestingly, government statistics suggest that some medical specialists have incomes that are outrageously high. I am not disputing those statistics, but I do know that such high salaries are not earned by primary care physicians, pediatricians, and psychiatrists. On top of that, over the last few years, I have seen my spendable income drop. Also interesting: the figures I've not seen published are in regard to insurance companies' profit margins, which were already large and yet have constantly increased over the years. Neither have printed statistics spoken to the rapid escalation in health maintenance organizations, whose profit margins have also been increasing annually.

Shrinking Patient Benefits

The Health Maintenance Organization Act of 1973 legislated by Congress required health maintenance programs to provide a certain amount of coverage for psychiatric care. The original intent of the law was to make psychiatric care more available to patients by requiring HMOs to offer coverage for up to a certain number of patient visits.

Originally, the law stated that a minimum of twenty outpatient visits and thirty hospitalization days be covered per year. After time, however, the law has been changed to reflect diminished numbers. In fact, the minimum number of days has now become the maximum number of days that a patient can get covered by any HMO. There are isolated incidents in which, with increased premiums, those benefits can be expanded, but clearly, the original intent of the law has been distorted, turning a profit for the insurance industry while placing harmful limitations on the general public.

Managed Competition

Managed competition, as it exists today, has tended toward harming patients, exhausting physician time, and creating ill will on the part of both practitioners and insurance carriers, all while removing the responsibility of payment for medical care from the individual patient and placing it on the physician. Some might argue that these effects of managed competition have occurred only because physicians are mismanaging their practices under the new systems. In all practicality, however, doctors are not businessmen, and they were never intended to be. Doctors are geared toward responding to their patients' health needs. Further, if doctors thoroughly investigated the financial aspects of things first, very few patients would get the proper medical care. Therefore, it is only after the delivery of adequate medical care that the business aspects of the relationship should be explored.

Over the years, I have concluded that managed competition, in theory, seems reasonable. In practice, however, there really is no managed competition. There is only mangled competition with increased patient suffering, decreased quality of service, and the imposition of third-party individuals in the patient-doctor relationship—individuals who fiscally benefit from the chaos involved in these programs.

Other Problems with HMOs

The entrance of HMOs into the medical realm has posed a number of additional problems. HMOs determine the number of physicians that an organization needs to provide for the patients contracted for their insurance services. First, when the number of primary care physicians or specialists in a given HMO is reached, other equally trained and competent practitioners may be denied acceptance into that HMO. As a result, patients may be required to drive exorbitant distances just to see a physician enrolled in their HMO.

An additional dilemma is the issue of confidentiality, a particularly troublesome issue when dealing with psychiatric records, which are more sensitive in nature than usual medical records. Sometimes the HMO or IPA insists having access to all of an enrolled patient's medical records, and there is no control, by either the patient or the physician, over how those records are used and what rules of disclosure will apply.

Finally, medical students do not gain exposure to the range of patients they once did. When I was in medical school, a key ingredient in quality medical training was exposure to patients with a variety of medical pathologies. Through this exposure, we were taught to develop differential diagnoses lists. The analogy is, in medical school, we were taught that when you hear hoof beats, you think first of horses, but in the training centers, we were exposed to both zebras and horses. In short, we learned that the obvious diagnosis was not the only possibility.

Now, because of managed care, major training centers—out of their need to compete for patient numbers—offer discounted rates and have decreased censuses. As a result, there have been drastic cuts in bed occupancy, meaning medical schools like UCSF do not have the variety of patients they once did, and students do not have exposure to as wide a range of patients. Ultimately, then, today's physicians-in-training never see the complex cases needed to develop sufficient clinical skills, which, in the long run, again, might be detrimental to their patients.

My Colleague's Experience

Many years ago, a colleague of mine decided that private practice was no longer to his liking, and went to work for a local hospital in the department of psychiatry. The hospital was a network provider for California's largest HMO, Kaiser Permanente. When he started, my friend realized that there were areas of neglect within the system. Namely, he realized that Kaiser's psychiatric coverage was limited to acute, medically necessary psychiatric care. Further, patients labeled as chronically ill were not eligible for psychiatric benefits under Kaiser's program. A chronic illness in psychiatry—for example, schizophrenia, bipolar disorder, or major depression—is the equivalent of a catastrophic illness. Clearly, however, that was not Kaiser's interpretation, because as soon as a patient was labeled with such a condition, Kaiser would deny him or her further psychiatric benefits. Such denial is contrary to why most patients have medical insurance to begin with. All of us want to be protected against any expensive devastating illness that may come along, and we expect our insurance companies to help with those kinds of catastrophic events. As a side note, part of Kaiser's interpretation may have been due to the industry's general relegation of psychiatry to the role of medicine's stepchild. It is my belief that medical insurance companies have had a prejudicial view of mental illness for decades. Psychiatric illness and treatment has been seen as ineffective, costly, and a drain on the system, with few functional human beings emerging at the end of treatment. The fact that mental illness was not provided with the same coverage as other "physical" illnesses until the 1990s demonstrates that prejudice.

Clearly, with the advent of better evidence-based research delineating the biological basis of many psychiatric diseases and the proven effectiveness of new treatment modalities, psychiatry has gained credibility within medicine. Within its own ranks, prominent psychiatric experts in the 1990s debated the effectiveness of treatments. Dr. Thomas Szasz has long preached about the myth of mental illness.[14] Dr. Peter Breggin published his opinions in his work *Toxic Psychiatry*,[15] and earlier, Dr. E. Fuller Torrey wrote *The Death of Psychiatry*.[16] There were debates as to whether psychiatric conditions qualified as diseases with clear causes and definite possible cures. It's little wonder, with psychiatry not able to get its act together, that insurance carriers, Kaiser included, would limit mental-health coverage.

In 1996, with the introduction and passage of the Mental Health Parity Act, psychiatry's major conditions—major depression, schizophrenia, bipolar illness, organic brain conditions, and obsessive compulsive disorder—were required to be covered by insurance carriers on an equal plane with other physical illnesses.

In another area of his job, my colleague discovered there had been very little liaison work within the hospital, particularly between the department of psychiatry and the separate departments of obstetrics and pediatrics. He realized that pediatric and obstetrical patients had significant needs that were psychiatric in nature, however, and that it behooved him to get to know the pediatricians and obstetricians, and to facilitate increased sensitivity to the psychiatric needs of their patients. Following his initiation of closer relationships with such specialists, his hospital suddenly had far more referrals from Pediatrics and Obstetrics.

If looked at purely from the standpoint of the medical needs of the patients, this would be a desirable situation, both in the short term and in the long. Numerous studies have shown that the availability of psychiatric services to medical clinic patients reduces the return rate of those with vague somatic complaints to their primary care physicians. In fact, one Kaiser study uncovered such a pattern: patients seeking medical care for the wrong reasons, when the psychiatric aspects of their diseases are pursued, utilize other medical services less, even though their usage of psychiatric services may increase for a time. Therefore, the increased referrals that my colleague brought on, if looked at in terms of the patient's reduced need for pediatric and obstetrical services, would be seen as desirable. However, my colleague was reproached for his actions by his chief of psychiatry. Basically, the shortsighted head of his department saw only that he had increased the workload on psychiatry by creating more demand for their services than there had been previously.

That's because by this time the system had devolved into one in which the lesser the flow of patients between primary care services and specialty clinics, the easier the job would be for the specialists. Clearly, however, such a system creates a conflict of interest at the expense of patients. In this case, patients were denied access to care that would be helpful and perhaps vital to them. It was no wonder that such a disconnect had existed between psychiatry and obstetrics and pediatrics before. It was simply far easier on the physicians in these specialty clinics to deal not as part of a team but independently from other primary care doctors, decreasing referral work.

A Contradiction

The end result of the entrance of the HMO model into the medical establishment is a very interesting contradiction: the less efficient the system, and the less often patients are treated, the greater the profit margin for the corporation and its physician partners.

Yet More Interesting Changes Brought on by HMOs

- Cataract surgery, the treatment of choice, was less likely to be approved if a patient was a member of an HMO than if not contracted with an HMO, according to an editorial in the June 1997 issue of the *Journal of the American Medical Association*[17]

- Prior to HMOs, the average time primary care physicians spent with their patients in a private practice setting was twenty minutes. Now, the average amount of time spent is eight minutes.

- Managed care for cancer patients and patients requiring state-of-the-art therapies is an extreme problem. In regard to the latter, such therapies are more expensive because they are on the cutting edge and provide the greatest benefit, but, because there is still little experience with them, are easily labeled as experimental. It takes time for new treatment methods to become the norm. Therefore, despite their promise and demonstrated usefulness, these methods may be excluded by managed care companies on the basis of not being proven beneficial—but with the underlying reason being cost.

My Personal Experiences with HMO Intrusion

When I graduated medical school in 1969, the Kaiser Foundation Hospitals were widely viewed as a place marginal MDs went to practice medicine. Unfortunately, when I was in medical school, the only health insurance my wife and I could afford was Kaiser Permanente; therefore, my oldest son was delivered at Kaiser. There was not enough staff available on the weekend my wife went into labor, and she was poorly monitored. My son had a "high forceps" delivery and suffered anoxia, which resulted in brain damage, rendering him ultimately developmentally disabled, prone to episodic seizures and mild cerebral palsy.

It took years of multiple evaluations to clarify the extent of my son's physical damage. Often, his developmental delays were dismissed with statements like, "Perhaps you're overreacting because of your profession." One pediatrician even said, "My son didn't talk until he was four, and now he's in medical school."

That said, my wife and I never pursued a lawsuit against the hospital, feeling the possible monetary gains would not remedy the problem. Bad things happen, and you can't always resolve them with money.

The Kaiser Hospital System
Kaiser was one of the first attempts at managed care and certainly was a laudable early effort, but over time, has served as an example of how quality erodes and drifts to mediocrity, if not lower, when patient care takes a back seat to fiscal considerations.

Over the course of my forty plus years in the practice, I have had both personal and professional experiences dealing with the Kaiser hospital system. In this chapter, I will share the more personal vignettes; however, let me preface these various anecdotes by saying that I have a number of friends and colleagues who have worked within the system and that, they are, by and large, excellent doctors. These doctors, however, not unlike many others, have experienced increased pressure to see more patients in less time, to perform fewer procedures, and to use less-costly medications. Their income is frequently determined by how well they do all this, as opposed to by how well they treat their patients. In addition, these doctors have limited medications available to them, frequently forcing them to alter the medication that is best for a particular patient because it is not covered by the hospital's drug formulary (which is primarily dictated by cost).

I would also like to preface these stories by saying that my impression of Kaiser has improved with time. The medication formulary is still restrictive, but Kaiser is now a leader in health-care delivery. And, primarily because Kaiser is a physician-direct system, care for patients has improved.

That said, however, the following personal experiences, although they happened in the past, continue to be solid examples of the drawbacks of managed care systems in general.

My Father-in-Law
In the late 1980s to early 1990s, my father-in-law, a Kaiser patient, experienced several heart attacks. After each of these attacks, he was seen by various Kaiser physicians, but none of the attacks were

followed up with an angiography—a procedure in which doctors can take radiographic view of the blood vessels serving the heart to determine which arteries are closed and whether there is a need for surgical intervention.

Then, in 1994, while alone at home, my father-in-law had an episode of severe abnormal rhythm, resulting in another myocardial infarction (heart attack). His life was saved only by the quick actions of the paramedics who came into his house, found him unconscious, and immediately administered the correct treatment, including the use of paddles to restart his heart.

He was taken to a non-Kaiser hospital, where his cardiac function failed a second time. They again administered cardioversion (use of the electronic stimulation paddles), and after he was stabilized, transferred him to a Kaiser hospital.

Seven days later, he was finally given an angiogram, which revealed severe blockage of his coronary arteries. He required quadruple bypass surgery, however, Kaiser did not have a cardiac surgeon available. It wasn't until two weeks following his cardiac arrest that he was in surgery in a non-Kaiser hospital.

Post-op, Kaiser determined that follow-up tests, to determine the cause of his abnormal rhythm and the necessity of implanting a pacemaker to prevent reoccurrence of that abnormal rhythm, unnecessary.

My father-in-law was discharged from the hospital three days after his surgery. We fought with Kaiser to allow him to go to a nursing home, to which they reluctantly agreed, with the promise that he would be allowed to stay there for a week.

Two days after he entered the nursing home, a Kaiser doctor appeared and saw him for the first time. The physician did a brief, cursory examination that was clearly inadequate and discharged him from the nursing home that day.

Because of the poor post-operative course doctors had taken with him, my wife and I took him into our home for one month, and he had severe complications. He had bleeding that necessitated transfusion, and twice during the month that he stayed with us, we had to call paramedics to take him to the hospital to save his life.

Both times, Kaiser required that the advice nurse determine whether he could come into the emergency room before he could be treated. However, on one of these occasions, he was already semi-conscious when the advice nurse was called. My wife and I immediately determined that calling 9-1-1 was the only appropriate alternative to this uncooperative system. The emergency response only resulted in my father-in-law being monitored for a few hours in the emergency room, and then he returned to recuperate in our home. Since he didn't have an episode of distress while Kaiser was monitoring him, no corrective procedure was suggested. Although they had been developed at that point, internal cardiac defibrillators were never made available to my father-in-law.

Nine months after his bypass surgery, while driving alone in his car, he presumably had another cardiac arrest. He had the fortunate premonition that something terrible was happening and was able to pull over to the side, under a tree. He was found dead in his car about three hours later. This man was a wonderful, dynamic, productive, caring human being. He was an Episcopal priest who provided spiritual guidance to hundreds of people, and his death was a significant loss to humanity. Yet, at age sixty-two, through Kaiser's negligence, he was taken from us.

My Brother

In 1995, my brother, aged fifty-nine, experienced severe chest pains while working in his garden. His wife took him to a Kaiser hospital, where he was stabilized in the coronary care unit. Again, no angiography was ordered, but blood tests determined that he had had a myocardial infarction. He was scheduled to be sent home in three days.

I called the Kaiser physician as a relative concerned about my brother's welfare and health, and curious about the plan for follow-up studies. The physician was offended when I asked about an angiography, suggesting that if I wanted to be the treating physician, she would be happy to turn over my brother's care to me. Needless to say, I was outraged. I asked her why, when I was only inquiring about my sibling's health and asking for a medical explanation for their treatment plan, she was reluctant to give it to me. My brother was finally given some cursory, low-cost evaluation of his heart.

Later, at my insistence, he sought a second opinion from a private cardiologist in whom I had a great deal of faith. This physician outlined, on paper, a plan for adequately assessing my brother's cardiac condition, and my brother took that to Kaiser. An angiography was done, and significant cardiac-tissue damage was found. Sophisticated tests that determined his need for an operation were also done, and five months after his myocardial infarct, he had quadruple bypass surgery. I suspect that only because I was a physician, only because I persisted in my efforts to get him the care that he had a right to, and only because we had a very strong, reliable second opinion did he ever have the surgical intervention.

In his recuperative phase, however, my brother began to experience gallbladder problems. Again, with a great deal of prodding, Kaiser finally ran studies to show that he had significant gallstones, but then the surgeon quoted literature that was outdated to support delaying the necessary surgery to remove his gallbladder. He stated there would be a significant risk to my brother if the surgery were done within six months of his bypass surgery. Today, gallbladder surgery is an extremely refined and easy procedure that needs not tax the cardiac system, but the studies this Kaiser doctor cited were done prior to the advent of laser surgery and the refinement of surgical techniques that would ultimately be used on my brother.

Consequently, for six months, he had numerous gallbladder attacks, which I feel posed an even greater risk to his cardiac status than surgical intervention would have. Finally, though, my brother did have gallbladder surgery, with no problems and no interference with his cardiac recovery.

Such delays in the implementation of care to cardiac patients are inexcusable. In my father-in-law's instance, I believe it resulted in his death. In my brother's case, I believe that, had I not persisted, he, too, might be dead.

In light of these two incidents, it was interesting to me to realize that when patients sign up for the Kaiser program, they sign an agreement not to resort to the courts in instances they believe to be malpractice. They also sign an agreement that binds them to an arbitration process which would make it extremely difficult to find an attorney who would sue Kaiser Foundation Care. Most Kaiser patients, if you ask them, do not remember signing such an agreement.

Since Kaiser hospitals are self-insured, the arbitration process, by definition, results in much lower awards to patients in cases of malpractice. In addition, according to the patient agreement, one of the three arbitrators in the case has to be an attorney employed by Kaiser. Further, while another can be an attorney selected by the patient, the third has to be an attorney agreed to by Kaiser. How much is that deck stacked against the patient? How significantly skewed in Kaiser's favor is the entire setup?

Unfortunately, these agreements have allowed Kaiser to get away with practicing poor quality medical care over many years. However, as I stated earlier, I think the system has improved.

My Mother-in-Law
After my father-in-law's death, his wife—my mother-in-law—lived on and took care of herself. One day, while hurrying to get inside the market before it closed, she tripped and fell, severely fracturing her

right wrist and breaking her right kneecap. If she had not had Kaiser care, she would have immediately gone to an emergency room. There, a surgeon would have been called, and he or she would have performed the correct orthopedic procedure within twenty-four hours.

Kaiser's response was as follows: she was admitted to the emergency room, where her wrist was put in a cast and her knee was put in a brace. She was not seen by an orthopedist in the emergency room; instead, she was sent home and told to return the next day to see the orthopedist.

The next day, her fingers and hand were blue for lack of circulation. Despite the surgeon's attempts to get her in for surgery, it could not be scheduled until eight days after her injury. She was sent home in excruciating pain with a severely broken wrist.

The night before her surgery, she was readmitted to the hospital because she had developed thrombophlebitis in her right leg, which had kept her from walking during this entire waiting period. Thrombophlebitis, or blood clots, is a complication that could be potentially life-threatening, as one of the clots in her leg could dislodge itself and travel either to her heart or to her brain. Clearly, however, it was the delay in her care that resulted in this condition.

In surgery, four steel pins had to be placed in her wrist, and the wrist needed to be stabilized both internally and externally. She looked something like an erector set when she came home from the hospital.

In terms of her post-operative care at home, Kaiser would only provide a wheelchair, which was ludicrous. She could only use her right arm and left leg to move the chair, which if I calculate correctly, meant that her only ambulating would be to move in circles. (If you move the right wheel and cannot move your leg, the chair turns in a circle.)

Before her surgery, the only help she received to keep her in some sort of reasonable condition was provided by my wife who was a

R.N. It was my wife who diagnosed the thrombophlebitis. It was my wife who bathed and cared for her mother daily. Had we not been a medical family looking out for the needs of our relative, however, God knows what the result would have been.

A Huge Contrast in Care

In contrast to those I have known who've gone through the Kaiser system, my mother, at age eighty-two, went to a non-Kaiser hospital when she experienced a myocardial infarction. As mentioned previously, my mother was a very strong-willed, stoic individual. Late in the day that she had her heart attack, I called her to ask how she was. She said that she'd had chest pain all day, but thought it would be going away soon. I could tell by the tone of her voice that she was in pain, and I could tell by her description of the pain that it was serious. I immediately told her and my father that they had to get in the car and get her to a hospital.

They chose to bring her to the hospital that was closest to me, about forty miles from their home. Her insurance coverage was Medicare, with a supplemental health plan to cover expenses beyond what Medicare would. Within twelve hours after her myocardial infarction was diagnosed, she had an angiography, which clearly showed the damage to her heart and the amount of blockage to the coronary arteries. Within twenty-four hours, she was in surgery, and although her age, high blood pressure, and general health condition were risk factors, she did very well postoperatively. She remained in the hospital ten days, had excellent post-coronary care and instruction, and saw excellent results due to the quick intervention and prompt attention that had been given to her problem.

Her cardiologists, Dr. Young and Dr. Strunk, had had no hesitations about doing what was best for her. They didn't have to respond to corporate fiscal constraints or worry about answering to some higher bureaucratic authority. They only had to be physicians and to treat their patient the best they knew how. Her surgeon, Dr. Hanna, responded the same way. He knew she needed the surgery and needed it quickly, and he gave her excellent care.

As mentioned, Kaiser has seemingly improved since the time of these experiences. In regard to the system as a whole, however, I sometimes wonder if things have improved or whether health care in general has deteriorated so much that we just now settle for less, allowing the insurance providers to determine the appropriate treatment options.

My Professional Experiences with HMO Intrusion

In this chapter, I would like to illustrate, from the standpoint of a physician, some of the problems I have seen with HMO intrusion into the quality of medical care. Most of these experiences occurred in just the last couple of years.

Economic Profiles

HMOs now maintain economic profiles on all of the physicians in their networks. Economic profiles show what services cost for the average patient walking through that doctor's doors; in turn, doctors are rated according to those costs. For example, the psychiatrist who delivers the least amount of services will have the highest rating with an HMO because he or she has cost the health maintenance organization the least amount of money. There is no quality care rating built into such a profile; the HMO looks only at the economics involved.

I was surprised several years ago when a list of the psychiatrists in my area along with their affiliated economic ratings showed that I had the worst economic rating with a certain HMO, meaning I had been the most costly to that health maintenance organization in terms of patient care.

Looking closely at the profile, I realized that very few patients I saw actually belonged to that HMO. However, one particular case stood out: a fifteen-year-old girl, who had come into the hospital in an acutely psychotic state. She had been previously seen by another psychiatrist, labeled schizophrenic, and treated with neuroleptics, but had failed to respond. Because of this and her parents' wish for another physician's opinion, I was asked to take over her care.

When I met her, I knew immediately that something about her previous diagnosis did not fit. She did not look like the schizophrenic patients I had seen in the past. There was something about her that was far more confused and organic.

Taking a very detailed and thorough history, I discovered that she had symptoms that were more consistent with systemic lupus erythematosus, an autoimmune disease that, in one of its rarest presentations, can mimic psychotic illness or schizophrenia. According to medical literature, a diagnosis of lupus erythematosus takes an average of ten years to make, and typically costs hundreds of thousands of dollars because of the multiple hospitalizations, medications, and lengthy hospital stays that occur.

In this patient's case, however, because of my perhaps serendipitous thinking, the appropriate laboratory studies and a consultation with a rheumatologist confirmed her condition right away. She was promptly able to receive the correct medication and her disease was brought under control. Now, many years later, she has had no recurrence of her psychiatric disorder, no rehospitalizations, and no need for ongoing psychiatric care, other than an occasional visit to my office to make certain things are going well.

Despite the fact that I diagnosed her disease correctly the first time, ultimately saving her and the HMO literally thousands of dollars on her medical care, I was seen by this HMO as its most costly and inefficient psychiatrist. The specifics of the case that caused my economic rating to be so low were not reflected in the data. All that was important was the expenditure the HMO had to make for her initial hospital stay.

It's alarming that such economic profiles exist, and that, in times to come, they will probably be relied upon for making doctor referrals (i.e., doctors with higher ratings would receive more referrals and those with lower ratings would have a more limited number). If that happens, it may well mean that the better physicians in the community would have fewer patients, because the figures used by the HMOs are often skewed, not reflecting the complexity of each medical diagnosis and treatment.

Spending Money to Avoid Cost

Another alarming case I had involving an HMO patient was that of a woman who had suffered for several years from depression. Another psychiatrist had insisted that she take one particular medication, to which she responded briefly but then continued to have depressive problems. I was asked to take over her care and provide a second opinion. Over time, I tried multiple antidepressants on her, none of which proved to be very effective. Her symptoms were consistent with depression, but there were also certain abnormalities in her presentation that made her situation unique.

For several years, the health maintenance organization resisted my attempts to get her a consultation from the University of California, San Francisco. They, instead, diverted her care to other consultants who did not have the expertise needed to help her with her problems. In essence, the HMO spent more money trying to find the least expensive method of dealing with her. And in the process, they caused her extreme anguish, prolonging her suffering.

Ultimately, after outbursts from me and her primary care physician to get her the consultation she needed, the HMO relented, and she was referred to an appropriate specialist. That specialist discovered that her depression involved a pituitary abnormality, requiring a different treatment approach altogether. It took *three years* after my initial attempts to get her the consultation for the HMO to respond and allow her the treatment she needed.

Further HMO Intrusion into Quality Medical Care

Case number three is even more painful for me to explore, since, every step of the way, I watched this woman suffer as she experienced abuse by her insurance carrier. Mrs. X, we'll call her, came to me approximately a month after she had been in a severe auto accident. She'd been stopped at a red light, with her seatbelt on, when a large truck had rounded the corner. Its driver, who was new, was not going very fast, but was unable to turn the wheel of the truck correctly. It crashed head-on into her stopped car.

She could recall the crash, but the details that happened immediately after the accident were no longer clear to her. She thought she may have struck her head on the windshield. She recalled being questioned by the police. At the police's insistence, she went to the hospital to be checked out to make sure she was not injured. She remembered being taken to the hospital without visible injuries, and being able to walk and converse with others. There, she was given a clean bill of health and sent home.

For several weeks after, she experienced nightmares, had recurrent thoughts of the accident, felt anxiety, and had headaches and neck pain. She was referred to me because her symptoms matched those of post-traumatic stress disorder.

This was a woman who had been exceedingly productive in her life. She had been a schoolteacher, and then received further education to become a psychotherapist. She had a relatively thriving private practice. She was a good clinician and was helpful to her clients. She was active in her church and in multiple outside activities, singing in concerts with her church choir as well as in individual performances. She was involved in her adult children's and grandchildren's lives, and she was physically active, often hiking and walking. But with her depression, all of these activities began to wane. She found her stamina dwindling, and her fatigue a burden. Even doing normal household chores had become difficult for her.

In my work with her, we addressed her nightmares, and she was able to work through the trauma. One recurrent dream that she'd had was of being in water and being swept toward a solid rock wall, unable to help herself. She would awaken just before being thrown against the wall.

Another recurrent dream was of being the protector of small children, and, despite her best intentions, the children would be harmed in some way, and she could do nothing to prevent it.

In their simpler interpretation, many of her dreams had to do with her feeling of helplessness to prevent the accident, its resonance with some of her past-life experiences as a child in Europe during WWII, and her need to see herself as competent and able, which indeed she is. The dreams had to do with her feeling a loss of control, which was a very important element in her life. She had felt in control of her life, her family, and herself in positive ways, but the accident had stimulated in her a fear of having that control taken away.

Even when her post-traumatic stress symptoms improved, however, her headaches persisted. Because of that, in consultation with her primary care doctor, I ordered an MRI (magnetic resonance imaging), a test that would provide a sophisticated view of her neck and skull, to check for any structural damage. Many years earlier, she had had pain and spasms in her neck, and was diagnosed with progressive disc disease. She was treated with a procedure called vertebral fusion, which was quite successful in eliminating all her symptoms. When the results of her MRI came back, they clearly indicated that she had, again, experienced trauma to her neck and that surgical intervention would provide a possible remedy.

A Fight for Surgical Intervention

Her insurance carrier insisted upon a course of physical therapy first. We found that physical therapy would relieve her symptoms for a couple of hours, but then her headaches and neck spasms would return, and her fatigue continued. She then began to experience symptoms that were progressive, with numbness, tingling, and, at times, shooting pain down her arms, which kept her from doing housework for any length of time, or making any other kind of repetitive movements with her arms. Even combing her hair became difficult.

We finally obtained a consultation for her with an orthopedist, who strongly recommended surgery. For confirmation, he referred her to a neurosurgeon, who also strongly recommended surgical intervention. The reports of both doctors, however, were cautious, saying there was no guarantee that surgery would relieve her symptoms. This was a reasonable stance for a surgery of this kind.

The insurance company, however, insisted that she see yet another neurosurgeon who was more equivocal in his report, suggesting that surgery was a possible solution but being even more cautious in his prognosis. He insisted that the patient undergo an electromyogram (EMG), a very painful procedure that measures nerve conduction. The test itself would not determine the need for surgery; it would only add a bit of data that would need to be weighed in the context of the full picture. When physicians make a diagnosis, they use the clinical symptoms, any appropriate lab tests, and any appropriate diagnostic procedures (such as X-rays or MRIs) to arrive at a decision. Most physicians were taught that "you don't treat a laboratory test." Clinical presentation is arguably far more valid in determining the need for surgery than this particular test. However, because her electromyogram did not confirm a delay in the nerve conduction, her HMO denied coverage of any surgery.

Now she was stuck. She had just finished a course of physical therapy and was to wait sixty days before starting a new course.

Except for muscle relaxants, which reduced the intensity of her pain temporarily, no medication had been effective at relieving her symptoms, and pain medicines tended to have devastating side effects. One pain medication in particular caused her to have visual hallucinations.

After some insistence on her part, she was seen again by the first neurosurgeon, and on this occasion he made a much stronger recommendation, saying that surgical intervention was needed. However, she was then asked by the insurance carrier to see a third neurosurgeon, who was a part of her provider panel. This man also made the statement that surgical intervention would "in all probability" be helpful to relieve her symptoms and suffering. By this time, several months had elapsed.

I wrote a letter in support of the need for something else to be done quickly. Time was passing, and her life was changing dramatically. Her psychotherapy practice was disappearing. Her singing activities were languishing. Her family was suffering. Her quality of life had been dramatically diminished.

However, even with an orthopedist and three neurosurgeons recommending surgery, the insurance carrier continued to resist coverage of this procedure, probably solely based on cost. Instead, they referred her to the University of California, San Francisco, to the Department of Orthopedics. It took several months for her to get an appointment and then several more to get a prognosis. The doctor examined her, recommended a few additional studies, and recommended review of her previous workups. After approximately four months, he concluded that surgery was necessary.

By this time, it had been almost two years after her symptoms had appeared and almost two years after the first recommendation of surgery, and the patient had still not had an operation. Where was the justice?

My sense was that, in her review by the insurance carrier, she had fallen into the category of an individual in a car accident who was trying to make money off of that accident. At no time during my contact with her, however, had she been focused on any remunerative benefit from the accident. She had only wanted her life to be returned. She wanted to resume gainful employment. She wanted to continue pleasurable activities. She wished for her pain to be gone. She had not, at any point, fit the profile of a malingerer, or of someone magnifying her symptoms so that she could somehow become wealthy from her injury. She was merely a patient who had suffered because of an insurance carrier's inability to respond to five separate physicians, all specialists in their field, who recommended the same specific medical procedure.

Over this two-year period, I had to continue to see her because she needed support in light of the problems that had not only continued but had also been magnified by her insurance company's inefficiency, greed, and shortsightedness. Her anger was contained relative to mine, as she expressed her distress to me.

The Outcome

Ultimately, this woman had the surgery she needed with a positive outcome. Her mood improved, her pain abated, and she was able to resume her professional work. She did not have a complete recovery, as her right arm still fatigues very easily if she uses it for manual work. The neurosurgeon told her that the excessive delay in having the procedure done probably influenced the lesser degree of her recovery. His analogy was that the accident placed pressure on her nerve tracts like a piano sitting on a carpet. If the piano is removed in a short time, the carpet resumes its original configuration. If the piano sits on the carpet for a long time before being removed, the carpet may never return to its original texture. This patient could have sued the insurance company. I don't know if she ever did.

HMOs and Experimental Procedures and Technology

My first contact with the atrocities of HMOs involved a consultation with a man who had a prolonged grief reaction to his wife's death. His wife had died from breast cancer, and he ruminated about his failure to secure timely treatment for her.

The patient and his wife had requested authorization from their insurance carrier for a bone marrow transplant, but were told it was an experimental procedure. Thus, there were excessive delays before the procedure was authorized. By the time she had the operation, the disease was too far advanced, and she died. Only after several psychotherapy sessions was my patient able to see that he had done all that he could, thus resolving his grief.

Around the same time period, several others had been in similar situations, also being denied bone marrow transplants and subsequently dying. Fortunately, in a landmark decision, the court awarded in excess of twenty million dollars to the family of just one of these deceased individuals.

HMOs, with their profit-margin mentality, will always be the last to approve new procedures or expensive technological advances. Therefore, some advocacy process needs to be a part of any future health-care system, to ensure the prompt utilization of new life-saving discoveries and treatments.

Effects of Changes on Health-Care Professionals

I once saw a young nurse in an emergency consultation. She had struggled hard to become a graduate nurse, having gone back to school after becoming a single mother. She prided herself in being an excellent nurse who was very thorough. Because she worked in a hospital that had had significant cutbacks in nursing staff, she didn't know where her assignments would be from day to day or what kinds of patients she would get. The number of staff members available varied from day to day to the point that they could not even count on being able to complete the surgery schedule.

On one particular day, she came to the hospital, met with a patient whose surgery she would assist, and briefed him on the procedure, which was to be simple arthroscopy of the knee. As she prepared him for surgery, she was suddenly informed by another staff member that no one was available to provide the laser support necessary for the procedure and that the surgery would have to be canceled.

She told me that this type of situation had always caused her extreme anxiety and anguish, but that, in this case, to make matters worse, she could see that the patient was already experiencing trepidation about the procedure. After learning it might be canceled, he seemed to be wondering what harm a delay might cause him. The nurse and attending orthopedist went to administration, pleaded for reconsideration, and asked them to find someone to provide the necessary support for the surgery. After about an hour, they were able to get into the operating room.

Effects of Stress

Because of the amount of stress this woman was under, her thinking became less clear. She began dwelling on all of the changes that had been taking place at the hospital and the resulting decline in joy that she received from being a nurse. She was constantly worried for her job and constantly worried that her patients would not receive the kind of care they needed.

Without her attention securely focused, she began to prepare the wrong knee for surgery. Then the surgeon started to operate. Obviously, both professionals were too preoccupied with the ordeal they had just gone through to provide optimal patient care. After a slight nick was made in the skin, the nurse realized her mistake. The orthopedist, at the same time, realized the mistake.

There was no harm done to the patient. There was only a very small skin incision, like that of someone who had bumped a knee and cut it. Despite this, the nurse was devastated. She felt exceedingly guilty. Her whole sense of herself as a competent, caring nursing professional had been challenged. She finished assisting with the surgery, but afterward, found herself unable to function at all. She went home and was exceedingly anxious. She became so severely depressed that she attempted suicide.

I saw her several days later. My diagnosis was depression, secondary to post-traumatic stress disorder. After reviewing all the facts, I blamed her condition on the extreme stress she had been subjected to on the job and felt that brief intervention and medication would solve her problems; and, indeed, they did.

I mention this story because it is a prime example of how the changing focus of medical care—away from the doctor/nurse-patient relationship and onto fiscal and administrative decisions—has compromised medical care. In this case, the change of focus almost caused damage to a patient, and it most certainly caused extreme emotional and psychological damage to a health-care professional.

I am sure, if I canvassed fellow physicians, I could come up with a hundred more examples of this kind. I do not believe that would have been the case ten to twenty years ago. This shift in focus, both in hospitals and physicians' offices, has been a terrible tragedy. It needs a remedy.

Problems in Caring for the Medically Indigent

On several occasions, medically indigent individuals on Medi-Cal have called me, asking to be seen. Because of my overhead costs, I try to limit Medi-Cal patients to a quarter of my practice, and perhaps I am somewhat unique in that regard, as many doctors will no longer take these patients at all. One such patient called and said that she had contacted over seventy psychiatrists trying to find someone to see her, and no one would accept her case. I had no room in my practice either and felt terrible. My secretary is very skilled at finding resources for people, however, and was finally able to locate an agency where this woman could get care. I can only hope that the patient followed up with the agency.

This example illustrates the reality in today's society that there is insufficient care for medically indigent people. Only when a situation comes to crisis proportions does care suddenly exist for them, and even then, the need for care is challenged. For example, if an indigent individual is depressed enough, becoming suicidal or homicidal or unable to provide food, clothing, or shelter for him or herself and his or her family, he or she will qualify for emergency hospitalization. At that point, the patient can belong to a psychiatric unit for seventy-two hours, or, if necessary, up to two weeks. The patient's problem will certainly not be resolved in that short a time frame. In addition, few resources will be made available to stabilize his or her condition. The individual will, in all likelihood, not receive treatment from a psychiatrist but from another type of mental-health clinician under a consulting psychiatrist. There will not be extensive therapy, never mind a cure, but there will be enough support to get the patient through the crisis until the next one occurs. This is the usual scenario for the medically indigent person who has a psychiatric illnesses.

A Typical Example

On one occasion, I hospitalized an adolescent for assaultive behavior. He was a young man with a very strange demeanor. Deaf from birth, he had violent outbursts and demonstrated other severe behaviors, including giggling to himself, probably as a result of some internal stimulation (e.g., hallucinations). He was fifteen at the time of his hospital stay. He relied primarily on sign language to communicate but had a low language level, and was unable to articulate his internal thoughts well, even with signed communication. His hospitalization came after his grandmother, who was taking care of him, awakened in the middle of the night to find him standing over her with a strange look on his face and a large heavy glass object held in a position to strike her head. She rolled out of the way, called the police for help, and he was taken to the hospital.

Interestingly enough, as the Medi-Cal reviewer was an ophthalmologist, the boy's hospital admission was denied. I called the reviewer to ask how in the world this particular case could be denied coverage. Why hadn't this case been considered a psychiatric emergency?

The reviewer's response was, "Well, he didn't hit her, did he? He only threatened." Ridiculous. Absurd. Prejudicial. In addition, certainly not in society's or the patient's best interest. Why would a fellow physician respond that way to an obviously anguished child, denying his hospital stay despite clear evidence that he was experiencing an emotional illness, displaying symptoms that made him a danger to himself and others?

After an appeal, the patient was allowed to stay for about a week, which, fortunately, was long enough for a physician to evaluate him, find that he was experiencing a psychotic episode, and place him on the appropriate medication.

Why This Happens

Classically what happens is that Medi-Cal runs out of money three-quarters of the way through the year. Then a message suddenly appears from them saying that costs must be cut. Here's how I translate that message: "Patient care must be compromised, and those people least able to defend themselves, least able to fight for their rights—psychiatric patients—are to be victimized."

This pattern of running out of money and thereafter cutting costs has occurred in California over the last couple of years. And the number of denials for hospital stays for psychiatric illness is only increasing due to budgetary crises and poorly informed individuals making decisions at Medi-Cal's administrative levels. These individuals are continually taking both the physician and patient out of the equation, making the decision process one of fiscal concern rather than of compassion.

Certainly, my experience with this boy's Medi-Cal denial was not an isolated one. At one point, to contribute evidence to a lawsuit that I had pushed the hospital to pursue with regards to Medi-Cal funding, I submitted over fifty cases in which I deemed the reviewer's decision for denying hospital care to people who needed it inappropriate. In none of these cases were we dealing with frivolous hospitalizations. They were hospitalizations that were *required* for the patient's benefit, but were denied due to fiscal constraints. The

State of California has changed how Medi-Cal is administered, giving each county the authority to regulate the spending of funds. That does not mean the system is improved, however; it now has different complexities.

Physician Turned "Enemy of the People"

When I was a college student, Heinrik Ibsen's play *An Enemy of the People*[18] made a great impression on me. In the play, a very interesting dilemma presented itself in a town famous for the curative value of its natural hot springs as well as for its health spas. The town's economy was centered on those springs, until suddenly a strange disease developed in the townspeople and in the tourists who had visited the town. The town's physician discovered that the source of the illness was the hot springs. The thrust of the story was how this physician went from being a well-respected member of the community whom people trusted to one whom people despised. In essence, because his discovery was seen as the cause of the town's economic demise, he was transformed in the eyes of the citizens into the "Enemy of the People."

Likewise, physicians today are being portrayed as the enemies of the people. They are depicted as being greedy, overpriced, wealthy entrepreneurs who have benefited from the suffering of the nation. In reality, however, I do not know any physicians like that. I know some doctors who live well, but it is not because they have exploited people for their own gain. I also know other doctors, like me, whose financial situations have changed dramatically over the last few years, due to the self-serving economic constraints placed upon them by the insurance industry.

In reality, it is the insurance industry that wants to make economic considerations the primary determiner of the delivery of care. The priority of physicians, established by the oaths they took as graduates of medical school, is to put quality patient care above all else. So who is the true Enemy of the People? The conflict is glaringly obvious.

Following Ibsen's analogy, the insurance industry is the large community. It contains a powerful lobby with far more monetary backing than the medical profession—or, in the case of the play, the physician. And just as the physician's care for the townspeople in the play threatened the economic stability of the community, today's practitioners who value providing quality medical care threaten the stability of the medical insurance industry. In the eyes of these large, profit-seeking insurance companies, then, doctors who take their Hippocratic Oath seriously simply have to go. Only those physicians satisfied with providing minimal medical care motivated by entrepreneurial greed will survive. The vast majority of physicians do not fall into this latter category, however, which means that if the trend continues, physicians will have to leave the profession in droves—and in their place, I fear, a new breed of physician/businessperson would emerge. Individuals on the covers of *Forbes* and those in Fortune 500 companies would replace the type of physicians who inspired me to go into medicine in the first place. And it would seem fitting, at that point, to throw out the Hippocratic Oath and replace it with the insurance industry's corporate golden rule that "he who has the gold makes the rules."

What a disgusting thought, both for me, in light of my personal convictions and the value I hold for myself as a physician, and for patients, who would have to see doctors who viewed them as nuisances to their guarantee of money. Patients would quickly be diminished to people for whom the minimal care should be provided, with the least quality and in the quickest time! I am sorry, but I would rather be a garbage collector—and I'm not besmirching garbage collectors, as long as they do not practice medicine.

Middlemen: HMOs, IPAs, PPOs, Etc.

Now on the horizon and being used by some physicians in private practice is an arrangement called capitation. Capitation is an annual contractual agreement that HMOs make with a physician or physician group, in which the HMO pays a particular set rate to have all of the medical care required by a given patient population provided for. For example, an insurance company may provide medical coverage for five thousand people within a community by contracting with an independent physician association that agrees to provide all of the medical care for that population at a particular rate. In ethical contractual relationships, the rate is determined by statistical analyses of the reasonable cost of medical care for certain groups of people, and the physicians within the practice group are compensated according to a fee schedule.

Capitated Contracts

Capitation as it applies to medical specialists has taken on the form of something called capitated contracts. The idea is the same. In a capitated contract for psychiatry, for example, the specialist, or in some cases groups of specialists, will provide, for a fixed fee, all of the psychiatric care for a particular community of people under an insurance carrier. Still using the figure of five thousand community members, perhaps the arrangement would be that each specialist in the group of providers is paid one dollar per month per patient, regardless of the services delivered. If the psychiatrist sees and provides care for only one patient who requires only one visit, he or she would be paid five thousand dollars. If seeing five thousand patients, each requiring one visit, the physician would still be paid five thousand dollars.

The Problems with Capitation

The obvious dilemma created by using a capitated system is that the less service the physician provides, the more profit is made. How can anyone keep his or her focus solely on quality medical care when the dollar is placed in such a high position of importance? Capitation is not kept a secret, but its availability in a policy is not advertised to policyholders either; patients have to ask their carriers whether it is a part of their plans.

I am aware of a number of entrepreneurial psychiatrists with capitated contracts who don't even see patients, but refer them to social workers, MFCCs, or psychologists instead, in an effort to increase their profits. I find this practice abhorrent. I am a good doctor, and patients come to see me because of my reputation as a good doctor. They don't come to see me so that I can "farm them out" to some lesser-trained mental-health clinicians. After all, I learned long ago that the contact between doctor and patient is as important in the relief of the patient's suffering as any medication given.

Capitation has been stated by many as the wave of the future. I am quite concerned about that wave. I am worried that it may be a tidal wave, and not just a ripple that I can swim through. I have been forced to look at capitation in my private practice to see whether it would be a viable concept for me. At this point, I am still undecided. I know of some contractual relationships in negotiation at this point with groups that I consider ethical. They are trying to arrive at a fair capitated rate that puts a limit on the amount of money I can make but also on the amount of money I can lose. That seems reasonable to me. I know of other negotiations that I want no part of, because the rates set are set unreasonably low. These other group plans appeal to some psychiatrists, however, who see the arrangement as a means to collecting a guaranteed income and making large amounts of money in exchange for providing very little care.

There was also a move to insist that specialist members of an HMO or IPA establish teams to bid on capitated contracts. This is a situation in which I would have no control over the quality of care practiced by the physicians they "put me in bed with," but would still share legal responsibility for the work of those physicians. For example, the HMO governing board could dictate that I be in a capitated contract with all of the HMO psychiatrists to provide care for their covered patients. If I want to continue to treat patients in that HMO, or to keep my current patients enrolled in that HMO, then I would need to form a treatment group with Drs. W, X, Y, and Z. But say that while I respect the work of Drs. X and Y, I feel the work of Drs. Z and W is substandard. Staying in the HMO would make me complicit with the work of two psychiatrists I believe are substandard.

Of course, I would have the right to say no and resign from the HMO, but I would not be able to continue to treat HMO patients or receive any new referrals from the group.

In insurance-defined programs such as HMOs, PPOs, and so on, the company defines who is accepted as a physician provider, and thus doctors have no control over the colleague they are associated with. For instance, one IPA I was affiliated with had defined as one of their child psychiatrists a physician with no official certification or training. He had defined his own expertise and experience, and the IPA had simply accepted it. On occasion, I had to consult on several of the same cases he did, and his lack of training was glaringly apparent. I complained, but to no avail.

The IPA also instructed physicians not to share any referrals or internal issues related to the IPA with patients; it was their perception of "loyalty" to the IPA. Wasn't the proper loyalty of the doctor to be to his or her patient? And that wasn't to mention their offense of First Amendment rights. The IPA would routinely lose bills they received from us for patient claims and then either tell our office staff that there was no need to rebill or ask for a tracer on the bill. Then ultimately, they would deny the claim for our not billing on time. Eventually, I resigned from the organization because it was clear that neither quality care nor honesty was a priority to that IPA.

HMOs and concepts like capitation, if they are the wave of the future, may turn out to be the cancer of the medical profession. They may devastate the ranks of good physicians by driving them out of medicine, and disease the industry's moral value system established by the Hippocratic Oath. They may ultimately lead to the death of medicine as I knew it twenty years ago, when the patient-doctor relationship was of the utmost importance and when physicians and patients alike valued the quality of medical care.

Tackling the Problems
I certainly do not envy President Obama or his staff in their attempts to tackle this overwhelming dilemma. They see escalating medical costs, and they place part of the blame on the physicians' failure to monitor themselves and stop unnecessary practices, and the other part on hospitals charging unnecessarily excessive rates for procedures. My hope, however, is that they also see the insurance industry for what it is—a large, very powerful group that, at this point, is making phenomenal amounts of money off of the public and off of physicians, and lobbying heartily to prevent change in the current system of health-care delivery.

The solutions to the current dilemma are indeed complex. In the next chapter, I will attempt to delineate the key elements necessary to maintain quality medical care and recommend solutions that may already exist in the models we currently have available to us. Granted, my views are only those of one doctor, but I am a doctor caught in the dilemma of having made an ethical pledge and now finding myself increasingly pressured to undo it. Hippocrates would be despondent.

Personal Practice Changes

I would like to describe how a typical psychiatrist office for worked when I began practicing twenty years ago. This is primarily in an outpatient setting, but I will also include some reference to inpatient work. In each case, a patient would be seen, for which a reasonable charge would be determined by the prevailing rate in the community, depending on the service rendered. A bill—including vital information, such as the name of the patient, the birth date, the address, and the insurance carrier's name, if applicable—would be prepared and presented to the patient to submit to his or her insurance company. The patient was then expected to pay the bill and deal with the insurance carrier directly.

A Different Era

My friend and colleague, Walter Harry Caulfield Jr., MD, once told me a story about his father, who had a surgical practice in western Pennsylvania. In those days, as a general surgeon, his father did a little bit of everything, from delivering babies to performing abdominal surgery to treating ingrown toenails.

Harry had decided to follow in his father's footsteps and went into medicine. Right after medical school, Harry had the occasion to help his dad with the business end of his practice. Times were tough. It was the end of the Depression, and people had little money. Very few patients had insurance.

Upon starting, Harry had looked at the books and then sat down with his father and said, "Dad, about one-third of your patients haven't paid you."

"I know, Harry," his father replied.

Harry went on. "Dad, don't you think you should send them each a bill?"

Without much emotion, the father responded, "Harry, if they'd have had the money, they would have paid me. If I send a bill, it will just embarrass them, and when they need me again, it might prevent them from calling and getting help. I don't want that to happen."

We don't have many physicians with that level of commitment to patients today, but I can't help but think we would be better off if we did.

The Paperwork Blitz

With the advent of business as a predominant force in private practice, much more detail had to be attended to—it had to be determined whether the patient was part of a particular plan and whether the doctor was a provider for that plan. If there was compatibility between the two, the patient was seen. Many HMO contracts required that the patient not be billed directly but make a copayment at the time of arrival in the office.

After a patient's assessment, in the case of psychiatric patients, the physician had to submit a review of the individual's psychiatric needs, in the form of a report, to the carrier. Those reports could be as short as one page, with relatively brief statements, or in excess of fifteen pages, with long, detailed lists of symptoms and other data. A diagnosis, obviously, was needed under both the old system and the current system. But when the paperwork was completed under the new system, it was submitted to the insurance carrier and not the patient.

Sometimes, before being seen by a specialist, the patient had to be referred by his or her primary care doctor, who served as a "gatekeeper" to ensure that unnecessary appointments did not occur. The gatekeeper physician, depending on the system, provides an estimate of the number of sessions the psychiatrist specialist will need to assess the patient and treat the condition. Usually, after the assessment is complete, a substantial amount of paperwork has to be submitted and a number of treatment sessions is requested. A reviewer determines if the request is reasonable and authorizes the additional treatment or suggests an alternative number of treatment sessions. With some systems, the response is universally a minimal number of patient visits and marginal patient care. Other times, the patient's insurance would have "carve-out systems" whereby a subsidiary business would agree to manage the mental-health benefits of the patient; under that system, a review of the patient's needs would have to occur before a referral could be made to a psychiatrist, and then the chosen psychiatrist would have to be an agreed-upon provider. Perhaps a nurse, a marriage, family, and child counselor, a psychologist, or another type of physician would carry out the review. A referral would then be sent to the psychiatrist and an appointment scheduled. This was somewhat cumbersome when patients were in life-threatening situations, as, for instance, suicidal patients cannot usually wait for days or weeks to be seen.

The use of carve-outs by health insurance companies is a method for separating specific services from general health-care services, and an unusual agreement and payment arrangement typically covers the designated service or services. Carve-outs may be offered by employers for prescriptions, dental or vision services, mental-health services, and similar benefits. And they may be provided to smaller employee populations or used to supplement employee benefits provided under a different insurance carrier. The benefit to the employer is minimization of the risk of catastrophic health-care claims; carve-outs allow the employer to share the risk with a third party.

Frequently in carve-out systems, patients have no ability to choose their doctors. Who they see depends entirely upon which psychiatrists were selected or signed up for that program. Unfortunately, there is no legislative stipulation that all qualified clinicians or psychiatrists be allowed to participate.

A Doctor's Dilemma

In my experience, the carve-out insurance provider more closely regulates what the practicing provider does than the principal overseeing HMO organization. Sometimes, a penalty is imposed on a psychiatrist who sees a patient before all the necessary paperwork is completed. The penalty is typically that payment is not authorized for that service. A doctor faced with a desperate patient asking for care would be in conflict with the Hippocratic Oath not to provide care, however, even if certain that that patient wouldn't be covered without the approval of the carve-out organization.

The Problem with Gatekeepers

Over time, likely because psychiatrists charge higher fees than other mental-health clinicians, there has been a move away from commissioning psychiatrists to see patients for their first visits. I am aware of one carve-out system, in fact, that mandates a patient's first visit be to a marriage, family, and child counselor—and therein lies a particularly interesting dilemma. As mentioned, because of the licensing procedures in the state of California, marriage, family, and child counselors are not given jurisdiction to make medical diagnoses. That's because, frequently, there are medical reasons for psychiatric illnesses. Many disease entities may show themselves via psychiatric symptoms but have a primarily structural organ-related basis, (e.g., thyroid disease, various manifestations of autoimmune disease, brain tumors). Therefore, some carve-out systems, as a result of excluding psychiatrists from the diagnosis process, have experienced significant financial liability for misdiagnosing patients and then attributing false reasons to their missing treatable or urgent organic conditions.

The same situation can occur in the gatekeeper system, in which a primary care doctor sufficiently sophisticated in providing physical diagnoses can refer a patient directly to a social worker or other nonmedical person. In this scenario, again, there have been a number of cases in which patients have been referred to specialists other than psychiatrists, the latter of whom could have provided more appropriate evaluations. Often, the result has been treatment delays and, in severe cases, devastating impacts on patients, including even death.

The Case of Mrs. Jones

Mrs. Jones was a thirty-eight-year-old woman who called me in desperation. She had been referred to me by a friend of hers, who happened to be a former patient of mine. She was requesting an appointment, and she was tearful, obviously depressed and anxious, and talking about being overwhelmed to the point of thinking about suicide. She happened to be a member of a health plan that contracted with the Independent Physicians Association (IPA) of which I was a member. She had called her primary care doctor, and his nurse had told her that a referral was being made to me, leading the woman to believe she could make an appointment with me immediately.

I gave her an appointment within one or two days, and when I saw her, I took a very careful history. She had been very content, both personally and professionally, until six months before. She then began to have trouble sleeping and felt anxious and depressed most of the time. She lost weight, her menstrual periods stopped, and she had no energy. Her first complaints to her internist resulted in a prescription for Xanax (an anti-anxiety medication), a referral to a psychologist, and a referral to an OB/GYN. She saw the psychologist about six times and was told that her problems were psychological—likely issues from her past and present—and "could not be related" to any physical problems. As such, it was recommended that she receive psychotherapy to discuss the stresses in her life. Further, the gynecologist told her that she was menopausal and needed estrogen, which she began to take.

Despite this treatment course, the patient did not improve. She felt an increasing sense of low self-esteem and functioned poorly at work and at home. In my first conversation with her, she struck me as being very depressed and anxious, but I could tell she was a very bright woman who had a good sense of herself. She did not reveal any major discontent.

"I love my husband," she reported. "I love my job, and I love everything about my life. I just don't feel normal."

She also mentioned that she had had skin rashes and that some of her hair had been falling out for several months.

I outlined a plan with her that involved starting her on antidepressant medication and getting her a more complete physical workup with a specific focus on her thyroid, even though she thought that had already been checked previously. I told her I had not yet received a referral from her internist (her primary care doctor), and she said would she check on it. She seemed relieved after our visit and scheduled a second one.

Later, I received a call from her internist, who happened to be the president of IPA, and he verbally chastised me for seeing her without authorization. There was no concern in his voice about the patient or about her depression and suicidal feelings.

His only worry, as he expressed it, was, "You had no authority to see the patient, and the IPA probably will not cover her appointments with you."

When I explained that her condition constituted an emergency in my mind, he said, "That is a problem in medicine today."

In addition, he objected to my recommending laboratory tests for her, and told me that when the patient had come to see him for a follow-up, he had eliminated four of the tests, ordering only a screening blood workup. Apparently, he had thought the others were unnecessary or too expensive.

Despite the internist's anger and unprofessionalism, I continued to see the patient. I explained to her my struggles with the IPA, but she said she wanted to keep her appointments, even if it meant paying for them herself.

One week later, I saw the patient again, and she expressed feeling better on the medication I had ordered. She said she was doing about the best she had been in about four months.

"I'm not back to normal, but I am about back to where I was when this all started," she told me.

I suggested she continue the medication while we awaited the results of the blood tests.

Several days after that, I received a telephone call from the internist, congratulating me for picking up on the patient's hyperthyroidism: she had Grave's Disease. No apology for his rude behavior; only some feeble attempt to cover his tracks by saying that in the ten years he had known the patient, he had not seen any change in her that would have made him think she was hyperthyroid. I was tempted to ask him if he was deaf—because she had clearly verbalized the changes she had experienced and they had not been going on for ten years—but I bit my tongue. I had to continue to work with this doctor, and with his powerful position in the IPA, he certainly could make my life miserable if I really pissed him off.

I still believe that self-serving financial concerns influenced the treatment of the patient in this case. Otherwise, why would the other physicians involved simply forget to order the most basic workup for a thirty-eight-year-old female with anxiety, depression, skin problems, menstrual changes, and hair loss?

Interestingly, this same internist has now published a list of qualities that make "a good IPA physician," and while quality care made the list, economic constraint is clearly stressed.

The Need for Balance

I agree that doctors have to be fiscally responsible and not order every laboratory test under the sun, but a balance needs to occur, and sound medical judgment needs to prevail over the physician's concern for his or her economic profile. Ironically, there is no quality-of-care profile, no assessment of the undue suffering of patients; only profiles on the cost to the IPA and complaints lodged against physicians. HMOs and IPAs claim that, in the future, quality-of-care assessment measures will be in place, but that economic measures preceded quality-of-care measures in the first place is certainly an indication of the priority of these organizations.

As mentioned earlier, when I began in practice, psychiatrists, in many instances, did not need help with billing. We could fill out the necessary billing form and hand it to the patient, who submitted it directly to the insurance carrier. Some psychiatric physicians are still able to operate that way, and a sizable percentage of my own patients have insurance that covers care in this manner, but many do not.

Now, the majority of the time, a psychiatrist submits a treatment plan to an HMO or carve-out, and then the case is reviewed by a nurse, who may or may not have psychiatric experience, or by a mental-health clinician, who may or may not be familiar with the medical aspects of the case. This frequently results in psychiatrists spending a great deal of time on the telephone arguing the need for care with a reviewer who, without seeing the patient, decides exactly how many sessions are needed. The reviewer sometimes even determines that the focus of treatment be medication instead of psychotherapy. And, of course, psychotherapy is certainly going to be the reviewer's choice above hospitalization, which is always the last resort, even if the denial of hospitalization subjects the patient to undue risk.

The Case of Ms. Smith

Ms. Smith was a forty-year-old, obese, blonde woman, first referred to me after a hysterectomy. She continued to have severe abdominal pain and, after eating, difficulty with nausea, vomiting, and extreme indigestion. I saw her for a brief time, fewer than five sessions, with no significant psychiatric findings except that, secondarily, she was depressed and anxious because her doctor could not find the reason for her pain. There was the continual suggestion that she had a physical problem which was yet to be diagnosed and thus required further study by her primary care doctor. I suspected that she had gallbladder disease, recalling teachers in medical school saying that typical persons affected by gallbladder problems had the four Fs: they were Female, Fair (light in color and often blonde), Fat, and Forty. I communicated with her primary care physician that I felt she should have a workup of her gallbladder status and that her degree of emotional distress suggested to me that there might be gallbladder disease. The family doctor politely ignored my suggestions. I suspect this was because they came from a psychiatrist.

For the next nine months, the patient continued having intermittent troubles and making visits to her doctor. She was finally referred to a surgeon who agreed with my diagnosis, and did an emergency gallbladder removal. After the surgery, the patient's pain was relieved, but she continued to have significant symptoms of depression and anxiety. Her primary care doctor tired of her complaints and started her on an antidepressant medication and on Xanax, a medication for anxiety. Periodically thereafter, her doctor increased her dose of Xanax repeatedly, until she and her doctor had a falling out. And, for unexplained reasons, her doctor, in a final prescription, gave her instructions to take 8 mgm of Xanax per day—four times the amount I have ever prescribed a patient.

The patient began taking this dosage and then sought the services of another internist. Upon hearing the patient's story, the new internist immediately referred the patient back to me. When I saw her in my office, she was clearly alarmed by the amount of medicine she was taking. She was not taking pain medicine, as she no longer had any pain; she was no longer depressed and so had stopped her antidepressant medication; but she felt she could not function without the Xanax and was well aware of its addictive properties along with the hazards of withdrawal.

She was correct. Individuals have had life-threatening complications during withdrawals, including seizures, cardiac problems, nausea, vomiting, blood pressure changes, and more. The patient had tried to decrease her dosage on her own before seeing me, but said it had been extremely hard. She would find herself doubling up in a fetal position, trembling, and just waiting until she could take her next pill. I immediately contacted the managed care company that provided her mental-health benefits and suggested that she be admitted to an inpatient unit for iatrogenically-caused substance detoxification. This was an emergency, and I felt she required supervised care in eliminating this now dangerous drug from her system.

I was told by the reviewer, who refused to identify her own professional discipline, that the patient first needed to try to withdraw on an outpatient basis. I spent one and a half hours on the telephone (obviously uncompensated) trying to convince the managed care company to authorize the hospitalization, all to no avail. Further telephone discussions with the managed care company continued for several days with the final outcome being that I would try to help the patient withdraw by putting her on a schedule in which she would reduce medication dosages very gradually. The process required that she be on disability for several months, with reduced income, and devoid of the support she would have had in the hospital, all while going through the suffering of an uncomfortable withdrawal process, which could have happened more quickly and efficiently if done in the hospital. Of course, all of this trouble dramatically reduced the expense to the insurance intermediary, by putting the financial burden and risk on the patient and on me as her physician.

Because of the problems with managed care, both the American Psychiatric Association and American Psychological Association have established hotlines that clinicians can call to complain about problems they have encountered. Since then, literally hundreds of examples of abuses of quality of care have been reported. In fact, because of the large call volume, it is not unusual for me to spend twenty minutes waiting on the phone to talk to a reviewer. On one occasion, it took longer. And this is all time away from further delivery of care. Time that cannot be charged for, and time that has made clinical practice far more complex.

A Reviewer Tells All

A nurse I know who'd had years of experience in psychiatry and medicine was once a reviewer for an insurance program. I will not identify that program, but most people would recognize it. Its slogan, "Don't leave home without it," is certainly misleading when it comes to the delivery of medical care. From the description by this reviewer, your life might be in jeopardy if you left home with it, or, for that matter, even stayed with it at home.

In the time she worked for this company, the nurse reviewer's performance was judged on the number of requests for specialty services she denied. There was, in essence, a quota system. Nurses who approved too many requests for specialty care were penalized or chastised, and when their approval rate became too high, they could possibly be terminated.

This woman, an older nurse, was appalled that she both she and the affected patients had to contend with this kind of treatment. After only a few months on the job, she quit, due to her ethical dilemma.

Again, the motivator for the reviewer's job was the monetary profit of the company. What this nurse was asked to do had little to do with patients' needs and all to do with the company's profit-loss statement and the value of their shareholders' stock.

This same reviewer stated that quality was never directly discussed with her as an issue, but said that she not only had a quota for the expected number of denials on claims but also a bonus if she exceeded the quota.

Billing Challenges

I now require a full-time billing person in my office to keep up with the paper flow. That person, depending on his or her training and background, can cost as much as 10 to 50 percent of my office income. Recently, I looked at the figures and found that the billing person's income would exceed mine in terms of take-home pay over the next year. Part of the reason for this is that I, like most physicians, am inundated with the need to have computerized systems. There is a requirement, by some carriers, that you have an electronic billing system, which allows you to submit bills over the Internet. Many doctors are not computer literate and certainly could not do that billing themselves. And even those who are computer literate may not have time to be involved with the myriad of medical billing systems available and their unique complexities, the logistics of which could take over that function of the practice. If there was a system whereby one set of paperwork was required with one uniform card for each patient and one central billing location, then the current complexity would be reduced dramatically. Doctors consequently have to pay billing specialists, who are able to demand higher and higher salaries as the need for their services rises.

Recently, one of my office staff called the claims department of an insurance company to tell them we had submitted a number of claims and were awaiting the return of income from those claims. My employee was told was that it did not really matter whether all of the information was correct on the claim or not. Regardless of how well my secretary did her job, 50 percent of the claims were automatically returned. The insurance company spokesperson said this was standard operating procedure.

There should be a change in the law to hold these carriers more accountable, as the ramifications of these practices are clear. When only half of the claims are returned, the insurance carrier can then hold onto the money, which rightfully belongs to the provider or the patient, for a longer time. Even if they ultimately approve the claim on resubmission, they have had an interest-free loan of that money until that occurs. The more that they can create a problem in the payment of billing, the more profit there is.

In other situations, claims reviewers have actually been told to "lose" a certain number of claims. Yes, a number of physicians and patients resubmit such claims; however, according to the estimate of a patient I have seen who worked as an insurance reviewer, well over 10 percent of people become so frustrated with the system they end up paying the costs of the "lost" claim out-of-pocket, and never rebill their insurance carrier for the charges, which they have been paying premiums to cover. The obvious result is the corrupt increase of the profit margin of the company.

Many of the commercials on television opposing health-care reform are sponsored by the insurance industry. These commercials emphasize the need for the patient and doctor to have control of health care and claim that the current system is working. In reality, however, it seems that the only facet of the health-care delivery system that is working, from my experience, is that of the bank accounts of the insurance industry.

A Call for Reform

We need some way to remove the middleman from the system and to monitor the graft and corruption, so that patients can get necessary care. Abuses should be detected and punished. For example, if a certain number of claims are "lost" or not responded to, there needs to be recourse.

For now, at least in the state of California, recourse can be taken in the form of a complaint to the insurance commissioner; however, those complaints largely go unheeded. The commissioner's staff, I am sure, is overwhelmed with the number of complaints that come in. They also have no investigative capability to follow up on all the complaints that come in.

Reform is needed. There is no question about it. The major question is: What kind of reform? Do we need a cumbersome bureaucracy intervening in the delivery of service? No. Do we need to eliminate the doctor as businessperson and allow physicians to return to treating patients, while implementing another type of monitoring process to detect abuses of the fiscal aspect of that care? Yes. Do we need patients to have free choice as to the doctors they see? Yes. Do we need a monitoring system to make sure that patients have access to primary care physicians when needed and specialists when needed? Yes. Do we need the elimination of non-qualified people in the decision-making process of medical care? Yes.

It is time for a revolution in medical care, and the driving principle behind it should be Ibsen's point: "What is really called for is a revolution of the human mind." This revolution should focus on maintaining the sacred physician-patient relationship, eliminating the physician as businessman, and returning to the Hippocratic heritage of *primum non nocere—first, do no harm.*

Brain Drain and Loss of Resources

Health-care professionals, principally doctors and nurses, have taken an oath to put patients' health interests above the business interests of a company. This makes them vulnerable to being exploited by business interests that do not share the same ethical concern. Unfortunately, human services is one of the fastest growing groups, in terms of employment opportunities, but also the area most vulnerable to the imposition of businesses and corporations. Some physicians and nurses, who seem to have forgotten about the priority of caring for patients, may have made successful adjustments to this change in medical ethics, but the vast majority of us remain in the same severe ethical dilemma. Take, for instance, the case of someone we'll call Ms. K.

The Case of Ms. K
Ms. K. was a fifty-two-year-old master's level nurse, who had been in the field of home health nursing for more than twelve years. When she consulted me for depression, she told me that was in her second bout of depression and had recently been put on disability because of her stress, fatigue, and anxiety. Her story, up until about one year before she saw me, had been one of a dedicated nurse with

significant managerial skills. She had previously worked as a regional manager for a large corporation in the home health field, and had been instrumental in the success of that company, building a thriving program grossing in excess of ten million dollars annually. She and the three other regional managers were all nurses with advanced degrees. They selected skilled nursing staff to visit ill patients in their homes and provide whatever care was deemed necessary by the patient's physician. In the midst of this successful venture, however, the corporation changed hands, and the new ownership decided that having professional nurses in managerial positions was a wasteful expense. They decided to replace the nurses with individuals with business backgrounds.

The woman's first bout of depression began after she was let go by this corporation without cause, and her sense of outrage, anger, and disappointment was directed inward, causing her to become clinically depressed and nonfunctional. She felt betrayed, unappreciated, and totally tricked by the new corporation.

She was successfully treated by another psychiatrist and was able to find a job with a new company. Depression crept back in, however, as she began work and got the feeling that her new corporate employer was going to recreate history. As she built the business of her new company, she became increasingly distressed by the sense that her work would not be appreciated and that there was no security in doing a good job. Still, she continued doing a good job and was making money for the company. Then, when her primary care doctor put her on temporary disability for two weeks, due to stress, history did repeat itself. Her company illegally dismissed her, obviously as a short-sighted way to save money, not appreciating the fact that she was the reason the business was succeeding.

I saw Ms. K in weekly psychotherapy sessions and provided her with antidepressant medication. Sometimes the work of therapy is validating the reality of a patient's perception and acknowledging her right to be distressed and enraged by the events of her life. This was the case with this patient, and with weekly therapy, her depression lifted. She was able to move ahead with her life and find another nursing position with a company that valued her.

Health-care professionals, principally doctors and nurses, have taken an oath to put patients' health interests above the business interests of a company. This makes them vulnerable to being exploited by business interests that do not share the same ethical concern.

The Future of Managed Competition

Medicine has, in the past, had teamwork and trust—trust between doctor and insurance industry, trust between patient and insurance company, and ultimately trust between patient and doctor. But that is no more. Coordination among the primary care doctor, family practitioner, general practitioner, pediatrician, internist, and specialist, all working together to try to determine what is wrong with a patient, synchronizing their efforts for the patient's good—none of this seems to exist today, and it certainly will not exist in a future of managed competition. All that will exist is a climate in which primary care doctors refer as many patients away from themselves as possible, as it will not be in their best financial interests to do otherwise. Specialists will also see patients as little as possible, since the fewer patient hours they spend, the more money per hour they make.

In such an environment, there will be little risk of overextending the primary care doctor; there may, however, be an issue of overextending the specialist. That's because, while the primary care physician and his or her staff are concerned with a patient's overall health, providing medical education and coordinating all of the necessary health services, specialists and their staff members manage the more specific needs of a patient.

In the idea medical environment, each member of the medical treatment team has a role, and there is an emphasis on quality, coordinated care. The general public needs to be aware of the implications of a breakdown of this medical team as a result of managed competition. Managed competition stresses the teamwork involved in the financial aspects of things, but not that involved in managing the clinical aspect—and they fail to see that there may be a clear incompatibility of those two aims. So, as the demise of professional basketball is caused by the emphasis on one player versus another, rather than on the team working together to success, the demise of medicine is caused by the seeming emphasis of one doctor competing against another, rather than on various healthcare providers working together for the patient's welfare.

Dr. M

Dr. M was a long-time psychiatrist in the county where I practice. For years, Dr. M primarily did hospital work and was an expert in one particular psychiatric treatment modality. Because of his unique skill, he was referred patients from all over Northern California. Obviously, his practice was very busy and, I would assume, financially lucrative for a number of years.

As managed care made its way into the community, however, and he began to feel the invasion of the insurance industry in his patient contacts, he began to assess whether he wanted to continue the practice of medicine, despite the fact that he had many years of professional work ahead of him. Unlike a number of doctors, Dr. M did not join a cornucopia of HMOs. He did not need to; they came to him, and he enrolled in enough for his subsistence.

Despite the fact that his practice remained busy, he found the ethical dilemma of revealing too much material to third-party payers very, very difficult. Greatly admired by colleagues, he had served on multiple organizations, been on a number of influential committees within the county, and acted as medical director of a hospital. He had excellent clinical acumen and was even one of the few selected by the

Board of Quality Medical Assurance to examine other physicians for their fitness to continue in the practice—a position that meant he was held in quite high esteem.

But suddenly, with about three months' notice to his patients and to the rest of the medical community, he prematurely retired and decided to go back to college to pursue degrees in English and philosophy, subjects that had always interested him. Financially, he did not have to worry, and ethically, the moral climate of the profession was becoming more burdensome than he could tolerate. Consequently, he left.

Dr. B

Dr. B has been one of my colleagues and friends for the past forty-five years. He is a man in his early seventies; he has three children, all attending private universities or graduate schools. Despite the fact that Dr. B would like to consider retiring, he really cannot afford to do so. He is one of the most skilled clinicians and astute psychiatrists I have ever known and a man that I probably admire more than anyone else in the field.

Recently, in discussions with him, I discovered that his practice, which in years past had always been busy, was now very empty. He had observed the invasion of the patient-doctor relationship by third-party payers early on in the process and refused to sign up for any HMOs or organizations at that time. Doing so would have required him to compromise his ethical position in patient care. He chose instead to rely on the idea that his reputation would bring him patients and that the quality of his work would speak for itself. His ideals were laudable but not practical, since the general public, although they complain about HMOs, do little to alter their existence. Consequently, as time has passed, my friend has found himself missing from insurance lists and devoid of referrals, unable to be seen in the industry to the fullest of his clinical capability.

Dr. B and I discuss practice frequently. I was not as astute as he was regarding the insurance industry's intrusion into my practice and I signed up for many plans. But I also, occasionally, get calls from people who are not confined to those plans. And since I have a full schedule, I try to send patients his way, not because I feel sorry for him, but because I know they will receive the best psychiatric care available. Some would say he is a dinosaur, but he is an honorable dinosaur. It is tragic that a man with his clinical capability now finds himself in a position of not having many patients, when thousands of psychiatrists far less capable than he are busy. He does not perceive his own situation to be tragic, and I certainly do not think his financial situation would be considered tragic, but there is tragedy to be found here. That tragedy lies in the fact that the public has lost a physician of his caliber because of a changing system that does not prioritize quality, and because those in the public and in the medical profession have failed to issue an outcry to change what is happening. Each of us has probably heard about cases of medical neglect caused by the managed care system, but we do nothing to alter the course of medicine, which is surely headed into a place where we do not want to go.

The Solutions

The key ingredient in any reform for this industry is a focus on patient care and medical benefit, not on political expedience or funding strategy. I am not advocating for socialized medicine, but I am advocating for some type of universal health care or a sophisticated combination of public and private sources of funding that utilize taxes, insurance premiums, and employer contributions. And I propose that any such reform in the United States should involve curtailing the role of the insurance industry from the reform process.

There is a conflict of paradigms that inherently exists. The overriding principle fundamental to HMOs and insurance companies is profit and company success. The overriding principle to medical-care providers is, or should be, patient benefit and providing state-of-the-art care to cure illness. Whereas people have compromised in the present economy to blend these two solutions, the attempt has been unsuccessful, with patients being harmed, the insurance industry making a great deal of money, the public becoming disillusioned with physicians, and the medical profession being compromised by the profit-motive mentality. As such, it appears that the principles that need to be incorporated into any plan for reform are as follows:

1. Per the plan first articulated by the Clinton administration, health-benefit coverage needs to be present for all citizens from birth to the end of their lives.

2. There should be portable benefits (i.e., a free choice of health professionals, including the ability to change providers without restriction and without exclusion for any preexisting condition).

3. Treatment decisions need to be based on medical opinion rather than cost.

4. There should be no restriction of access to physicians by "gatekeepers" (primary care physicians who financially benefit from stopping referrals).

5. Simplification of administration must occur with standardization of forms and billing and elimination of excessive paperwork.

6. Ombudsmen must be instated to serve as patient advocates when there are problems in the delivery of care. Highly trained nurses would be the most likely individuals to serve as ombudsmen because they have medical training and are bound by an oath to treat patients with compassion and understanding.

7. At the very least, major psychiatric illness should be treated on the same basis as other medical illness, with no punitive discrimination against citizens for having mental disorders.

8. Alternative treatments with demonstrated benefit (demonstrated, that is, by evidence-based research) need to be covered. Massage, some chiropractic care, acupuncture, and physical therapy are only a few alternative approaches that fall into this category.

9. Medical decisions and determinations of medical necessity need to be made by physicians, and particularly by physicians within the specialty that the patient requires, rather than by bureaucrats or physicians who have no background in the area in which they are asked to make a determination.

10. Confidentiality and patient privilege need to be guarded, and a legal penalty imposed when there is a violation of either.

11. There should be mandatory inclusion of physicians in planning benefit policies and in reviewing benefit plans and their functioning.

12. The profit motive of the intermediate administration needs to be reduced, if not eliminated. In this area, we must look to different countries for guidance (e.g., Germany, Sweden, Singapore, and England) and cull out the best of those systems—areas where those countries provide better for their citizens than is provided by our insurance-driven system. (Currently, administrative costs are driving up medical costs, not physician or other health-care worker fees.)

13. Federal standards need to be established for health insurance coverage. No state should be allowed to dip below those standards, although states could set standards that exceed the federal standards.

14. An effective appeals process, to guard against unreasonable program interference in patient treatment or in the doctor-patient relationship, should be set up as part of the law, with administrative accountability built in. Currently, there is no provision to penalize HMOs or others who have caused harm to patients without excessively long and costly legal battles.

15. Establish a team directed by a health-care czar—analogous to the federal reserve chief—with powers to dictate where health-care dollars are focused.

16. Currently, the renewal of the Hippocratic Oath does not require continuous monitoring of one's ethics and professional values. Doctors are only required to reactively review ethical principles—that is, they are only required to review them when they get into trouble. Instead, ethics renewal should be done on a proactive basis. There should be a renewal of the Hippocratic Oath every five years, with required updates of training. The principal to be enforced is ethical humanitarianism with evidence-based health care.

A Call for a New Direction

As a consumer and a physician, I have been able to glean information regarding the health plan proposals by the president and other proposals before Congress, and they basically put life-or-death decisions in the hands of non-medically trained people. Gatekeeper systems are frequently carried out by clerks or nurses working under strict guidelines laid down by insurance companies, or some other profit-motivated structure which signs their paychecks.

My perception is that the American Medical Association is so tied to big business and vested interests that its health-care reform proposal would be compromised and ineffective, keeping in place the corruption of the insurance industry.

A middle ground is needed, which preserves the right of patients and their selected physicians to determine treatment, while ensuring that health-care plans do not continue to reap billions of dollars in profit from the wallets of the sick citizens of the United States of America.

I recall watching the Obama inauguration and suddenly becoming tearful and overwhelmed with positive emotion. As a child, the son of a military officer, I attended many parades and took pride in being an American, and I adhered to the values of our country. It had been many decades since I had felt that pride and hope for the future. I feel it again under President Obama's leadership.

President Obama courageously pursued passing health-care reform that would limit the influence of insurance carriers on the delivery of health care. The Patient Protection and Affordable Care Act was passed in March of 2010. I view it as one of the first major steps to solving our health-care crisis and providing universal health care for all United States citizens. The United States is the last of the developed countries in the world that does not provide universal care for its citizens.[19] This reform is being challenged by the Republican sector of Congress for several reasons, but I believe that the real issue is whether the United States is brave enough to take the stand that health care is a right of our citizens; a large number in our country believe it is a privilege, and these people take the position that the government should not be in the position of directing medical care. I believe that it is better for the government to do it, as it has with Medicare, Medicaid, and medical care for the military, than for the present profit-motivated insurance industry.

Health-care reform would potentially give coverage to millions of uninsured people. The total cost remains unclear, but the direction is positive: there will be no denials for preexisting conditions, health care will be more affordable, high-risk pools will be established, Medicaid will be expanded, and fees will be limited. This will be the first major step to providing care for all our citizens and taking the control out of the hands of the insurance parasites.

Epilogue

As the values of our society and our world have changed, there has been a great deal of commentary about those changes being to the detriment of mankind. Thus, I believe the erosion of the ideals in the Hippocratic Oath parallels the erosion of many similar ethics in humankind in general. However, the necessity of the oath's inherent value continues unchanged. The tragedy is that medicine as a whole has not recognized that necessity, and thus has also not recognized the need to uphold, reinforce, and educate others about the tenets of the oath.

Subtleties within the oath have been altered as society's values have altered. Variations have occurred over time. For example, prohibition against abortion and surgery have been dropped as scientific knowledge has advanced and as societal morals have changed. However, the two basic premises of the oath that appear to be inviolate are to (1) do no harm to patients and (2) put the patients' medical needs above all else. The substance of the erosion of these principles, as discussed, is that the needs of the larger group as well as fiscal considerations have become more important than all else.

It has become clear to me that not keeping our priorities and values in order is one of the difficulties of being human. We sometimes allow personal acquisition and greed to determine behavior, motivation, and moral stance. A clear demonstration of that exists in medicine with HMO presidents making outrageous salaries while preaching cost-containment for patients. Some CEOs of health maintenance organizations make salaries of $700 million per year, while, at the same time, on the front line, a lifesaving procedure is being denied because it does not fall within the range of the patient's insurance benefit. I am not sure how individuals at the heads of these corporate structures can sleep at night or live with themselves in the context of what they have done to increase the suffering and health deterioration of the general population.

Trust

Since the erosion of the ideals in the Hippocratic Oath parallels the erosion of ethics among humankind in general, models outside of medicine are certainly important in looking at the erosion in this industry. The economist, Francis Fukuyama, has written a book titled *Trust: The Social Virtues and Creation of Prosperity*.[20] In that book, he encapsulates certain premises that I think are important regarding medicine today. One premise is that a building block of the success of any workable economic system is the establishment of lines of trust throughout the system's hierarchy. He gives examples of workers in Japanese companies who trust their bosses, whose bosses trust their superiors, whose superiors trust the board of directors, and whose board trusts the CEO. Obviously, I have simplified the process, but the main idea is that the lines of trust are there, and that they result in economic success for the company.

Within medicine, we now face a system in which patients do not trust their doctors. Frequently, patients also do not trust their health maintenance organizations or insurance carriers. Certainly, doctors do not trust the HMOs. Insurance companies do not trust the physicians. Ancillary staff do not trust the companies they work for, for fear of seeing reprisal or being laid off without adequate notice.

Earlier in this book, I made reference to the fact that one of the failures in my personal life was that I may have responded at times like I was more married to medicine than I was to my spouse. To carry that analogy further, the foundation of any solid marriage is trust—trust that the relationship is built on a partnership, trust that the partners together will solve problems, and trust that there will be no illicit relationships outside of the marriage that will undermine the marital harmony.

Patient confidentiality must be respected in the same ways as the vows of matrimony. Third-party interference that undermines the doctor-patient relationship should not be tolerated. Illicit relationships between the patient and the third party, or between the doctor and a third party, should not be tolerated. A prime example of an illicit relationship that does exist is capitation, especially capitation that exists without the patient's knowledge and puts economic issues above the primary needs of the patient.

As I have stated, within medicine, as it presently exists, there is a malignancy of mistrust. For the United States to reestablish a solid medical model for all of its citizens, this malignancy must be removed. Like a marriage, the doctor-patient relationship needs to be sacrosanct, inviolate, and come above all else.

A Move toward National Health Care

As someone who, in the past, felt that national health insurance was not the answer to medical care, I have turned 180 degrees to now believe it is the only solution to our crisis in medical care. In my experience, one of the most efficient systems and one that allows the best care for patients, is Medicare, particularly when it exists as a secondary insurance to cover expenses beyond the scope of the primary carrier.

Otherwise, I am convinced, health-care coverage options will only continue to get worse. This week, I had two patients denied the medication I prescribed for them because it was not on their insurance company's formulary. These were not new medications, and they were indicated for their illnesses, but the patients could not afford to pay for them out-of-pocket. I also saw a nineteen-year-old male with his first psychotic break—a manic episode from bipolar disorder. To do even minimal treatment on him, I had to talk to a physician reviewer. I asked for visits consistent with the standard of medical care in the community. The reviewer stated that I could only have two visits per month to prescribe medication. By doing so, in my opinion, the reviewer was only authorizing malpractice. I appealed the case with the position that if the company did not alter its decision, I would resign from its provider panel. My conclusion after that event, and after looking at many, many others: Things are not better. They are worse, and all that is happening is that we are getting used to it.

The Russian author, Solzhenitsyn, has an applicable comment on the subject: "It is time in the West to defend not so much human rights as human obligations." I would expand that to include obligations to provide access to universal health care.

If Americans are to receive the health care they deserve, we need to demand change from the current corporate, insurance-controlled system. Physicians need to abide by the oath they took and provide for patients by upholding the principals of that oath. Health care for all our citizens is an issue of human rights and is attainable, provided we demand it and hold our elected officials accountable for universal health care. Other countries with fewer resources than our own have reached the goal that we should be insistent upon.

Endnotes

1. H. Ibsen, *Ibsen: 4 Major Plays, Vol. 2* (New York: New American Library, 1970).

2. *Oaths and Laws of Hippocrates* (New York: P. F. Collier, 1910).

3. *Oath of Maimonides*, http://www.chiro.org/Plus/History/Persons/Oath-of-Maimonides/Oath-of-Maimonides.pdf.

4. *Declaration of Geneva*, http://www.cirp.org/library/ethics/geneva/.

5. *The Nightingale Pledge*, http://www.countryjoe.com/nightingale/pledge.htm.

6. J. W. Evans, F. Gensler, B. Blackwell, and C. Galbrecht, "The Effects of Anti-Depressant Drugs on Pain Relief and Mood in the Chronically Ill, *Psychosomatic*, Vol. XIV (July–August 1973): 7.

7. J. W. Evans and L. Glass, eds. *Mental Health Assessment of Deaf Clients, a Practical Manual* (Boston/Toronto/San Diego: College Hill Publications 1986).

8. W. Bogdanich, *The Great White Lie* (New York: Simon and Schuster, 1991), 186.

9. M. Grinfeld, "Rampant Fraud and Abuse of Medicare Funds Alleged at Community Mental Health Care Centers," *Psychiatric Times* (November 1, 1998).

10. R. Hackett, "Debunking Canadian Health Care Myths," *The Denver Post*, June 7, 2009, http://www.denverpost.com/opinion/ci_12523427.

11. B. Harden, "Socialized Health Care Analysis, Comparing Japanese Socialized Healthcare with American Free-Market based healthcare", *Washington Post* Sept. 7, 2009, http://www.gordonwaynewatts.com/FannyDeregulation/HealthCarePOINTS.html.

12. U. Reinhardt, "Health Reform without a Public Model, the German Model," *Economix*, April 17, 2009, http://economix.blogs.nytimes.com/author/uwe-e-reinhardt/.

13. M. Maddux-Gonzales and J. Mercado, "Primary Care Capacity in Sonoma County," *Sonoma Medicine*, Vol.63, No.1 (Winter 2011).

14. T. S. Szasz, "The Myth of Mental Illness," *American Psychologist*, Vol. 15(2) (Feb. 1960): 113–118.

15. P. Breggin, *Toxic Psychiatry* (New York: St. Martin's Press, 1991).

16. E. F. Torrey, *The Death of Psychiatry* (Berkeley: Penguin, 1975).

17. S. A. Obstbaum, "Should Rates of Cataract Surgery Vary by Insurance Status?" *JAMA*, 277(22) (1997): 1807–1808.

18. H. Ibsen, *Ibsen: 4 Major Plays, Vol. 2* (New York: New American Library, 1970).

19. P. Starr, *Remedy and Reaction: The Peculiar American Struggle over Health Care Reform* (New Haven: Yale University Press, 2011).

20. F. Fukuyama, *Trust: The Social Virtues and Creation of Prosperity* (New York: Simon and Schuster, 1996).

Suggested Reading

Altman, Stuart, David Shactman, and John Kerry. *Power, Politics, and Universal Health Care: The Inside Story of a Century-Long Battle.* New York: Prometheus Books, 2011.

Firedmans, Lauri S. *Universal Health Care (Writing the Critical Essay: An Opposing Viewpoints Guide).* Farmington Hills: Greenhaven Press, 2011.

Hunnicutt, Susan, ed. *Universal Health Care (Opposing Viewpoints).* Farmington Hills: Greenhaven Press, 2010.

Potter, Wendell. *Deadly Spin: An Insurance Company Insider Speaks Out on How Corporate PR Is Killing Health Care and Deceiving Americans.* New York: Bloomsbury Press, 2010.

Starr, Paul. *Remedy and Reaction: The Peculiar American Struggle over Health Care Reform.* New Haven: Yale University Press, 2011.

Williams, Richard Allen, ed. *Healthcare Disparities at the Crossroads with Healthcare Reform.* New York: Springer, 2011.

About the Author

J. William Evans, MD, is a child and adolescent psychiatrist in private practice in Sonoma, California. An "army brat," Dr. Evans spent his childhood in a variety of settings, including Northern California; Leavenworth, Kansas; Heidelberg, Germany; Arlington, Virginia; Saint John's, Newfoundland; and St. Louis, Missouri. After completing his bachelor's degree at Colorado College in Colorado Springs, Dr. Evans received his doctorate of medicine degree from the University of California, San Francisco, School of Medicine.

Board-certified in adult psychiatry as well as child and adolescent psychiatry, Dr. Evans has been in solo private practice for close to forty years. He has served as president of the Marin County Psychiatric Society, has been a board member of the Northern California Psychiatric Society, and has been a member of the American Medical Association, the American Psychiatric Association, the American Association of Child and Adolescent Psychiatry, the California Medical Association, and the Sonoma County Medical Society. Dr. Evans also has been designated a Distinguished Life Fellow by both the American Psychiatric Association and the American Academy of Child and Adolescent Psychiatry.

Dr. Evans and his family currently live in Sonoma, California, where he divides his professional time between his private practice and a public position as staff psychiatrist for both the Valley of the Moon Children's Home and the Sonoma County Juvenile Hall.

www.ingramcontent.com/pod-product-compliance
Lightning Source LLC
Chambersburg PA
CBHW031054180526
45163CB00002BA/833